About the Author

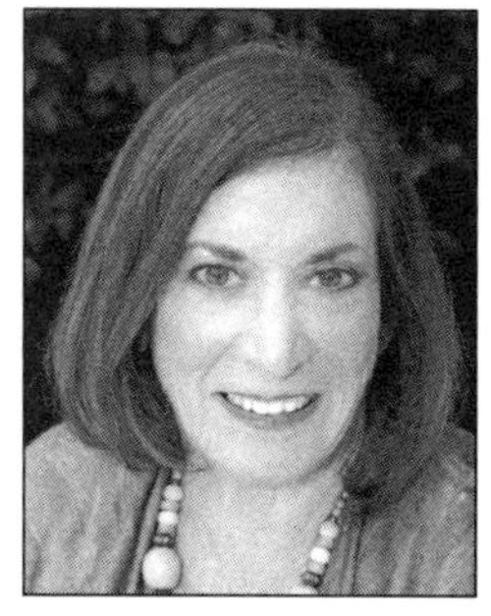

Dr. Gloria Kaye is a hands-on energetic healer who has been bringing relief to patients for decades. Her private healing practice has included children, professional athletes, celebrities, and even animals. She often works in conjunction with physicians and health care practitioners, and she has lectured on her approach to alternative healing to audiences ranging from medical students at the University of California, Los Angeles (UCLA), to medical personnel at the University of Miami.

In the 1970s Dr. Kaye did groundbreaking research on yoga as treatment for drug abuse. She earned her Ph.D. in clinical psychology and health psychology in the early 1980s with a dissertation on yoga—no small feat in a day when yoga was less than respected by the mainstream medical community. Part of her dissertation was subsequently reprinted in the Clinical Journal of Gerontology.

Over the years her healing work has been observed and documented by a number of respected physicians, and her practice has taken her to patients in the cancer ward at Cedars-Sinai Hospital in Los Angeles, California.

Though her home and practice are in Santa Barbara, California, Dr. Kaye travels extensively to see clients worldwide.

Sharing the Gift of Healing

Have you ever wanted to be a fly on the wall and observe how a true energetic healer works? This book is the next best thing. It puts you both over the shoulder and into the mind of a woman whose work has brought relief to many and is nothing short of phenomenal.

Gloria Kaye, Ph.D., has been practicing healing for decades and producing results so profound that medical doctors in a variety of specialties have become fans. In this unique book, she shares not only her stories, but also her techniques and the specifics of what she does to effect relief.

Her experience has taken her from the individuals she treats in her private practice and working with a professional sports team, to consulting with physicians and lecturing to medical students at UCLA. Not limited to humans, she has also had excellent results treating animals.

Her book describes, in depth, all of these experiences and includes:

- Detailed descriptions of techniques, including pendulum use, distance healing, and adjusting energy fields of the body
- Tips on self-protection
- Home remedies & health techniques
- Methods for partner healing

Healer's Hands, Healer's Heart is filled with case histories, Dr. Kaye's personal commentary, testimonials from clients, and verification from doctors she has worked with. It anchors anecdotal stories of healing with rigorous and fascinating factual documentation.

This is both an inspirational read and a how-to guide for anyone interested in this fascinating approach to health and well-being.

Healer's Hands
Healer's Heart

Healer's Hands Healer's Heart

In-depth insights, practical techniques and inspiring stories of success with non-traditional healing

Gloria Kaye, Ph.D.

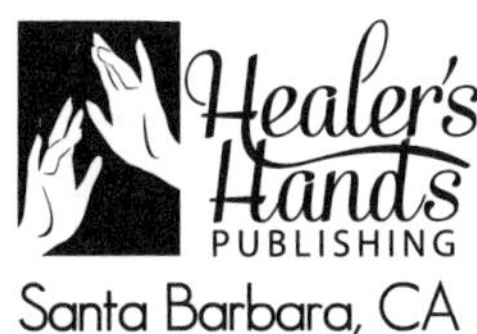

Santa Barbara, CA

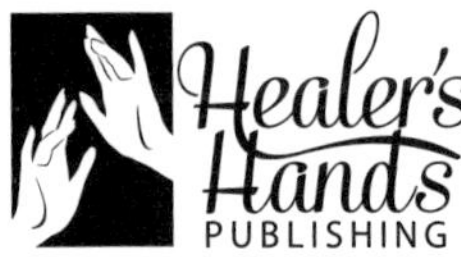

Healer's Hands Publishing
314 E. Carrillo Street, Suite 10
Santa Barbara, CA 93101
805-966-6104

This book is not intended as a substitute for the medical advice of physicians. The reader should regularly consult a physician in matters relating to his/her health and particularly with respect to any symptoms that may require diagnosis or medical attention. The publisher and author shall have neither liability nor responsibility to any person, or entity with respect to the information contained in this book. Every effort has been made to correctly report the flavor of the stories contained within; however, in many cases, names and places have been changed or deleted.

Disclaimer: some of the material contained in Part 1: My World As a Healer has previously appeared in an out-of-print publication.

Printed in the United States of America

Publisher's Cataloguing-in-Publication Data

Kaye, Gloria.

    Healer's hands, healer's heart : in-depth insights, practical techniques and inspiring stories of success with non-traditional healing / Gloria Kaye. -- Santa Barbara, CA : Healer's Hands Publishing, [2015]

        pages ; cm.

        ISBN: 978-0-9861247-0-9 (hardcover) ; 978-0-9861247-1-6 (softcover) ; 978-0-9861247-2-3 (eBook)

        Summary: This book is both an inspirational read and a how-to guide for health and wellbeing; not limited to humans, but treats animals as well. It includes detailed descriptions of techniques, including pendulum use, distance healing, and adjusting energy fields of the body; tips on self-protection; home remedies & health techniques; methods for partner healing. Filled with case histories, Dr. Kaye's personal commentary, testimonials from clients, and verification from doctors she has worked with, the book anchors anecdotal stories of healing with rigorous and fascinating factual documentation.--Publisher.

    1. Alternative medicine. 2. Holistic medicine. 3. Mind and body. 4. Mental healing. 5. Holistic veterinary medicine. 6. Healers--Personal narratives. I. Title.

R733 .K39 2015   2015901922
615.5--dc23   1504

Book Shepherd: Ellen Reid
Interior and Cover Design: Ghislain Viau

To my courageous, funny, loving
mother who lived
life with magnificent wisdom

Table of Contents

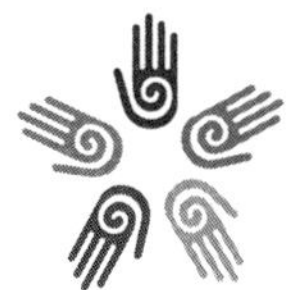

Foreword

You Just Have to Meet Her

What a privilege it is to be asked to introduce my mother. After all, she is the one who introduced me to the world so now it's my turn to introduce her. When I speak about my mother, I do so using superlatives. She is the most energetic, passionate and forward thinking woman I know. I often find myself attempting the impossible when I try to describe her as I struggle to convey all that she is about. After feeble attempts at trying to get the description just right, I resign myself to an exasperated, "Well, you just have to meet her."

Growing up, my mother was way ahead of her time. She looked for alternative forms of healing before the term "alternative medicine" was even coined. Homeopathy and yoga were far from mainstream. She was my secret to my own well-being, but the secret somehow got out. My mother was anything but a conformist. Today, I am so proud that she was willing to go against the tide. Her methods, her intellect and her compassion are sought out globally.

She amazes her colleagues, friends and physicians alike with her ability to heal so many serious conditions. Asked how she does it, she will answer simply that it is a "gift." And it is. If you asked her clients what Gloria does for them, with no exception, the answer is, "She gives us hope and comfort when both were unimaginable before we met her."

Here is the most amazing part. For a long time, many people, including myself, were skeptical of what we could not completely comprehend. We would demand to understand the "HOW" and the "WHY" and frankly, we would get in the way of ourselves. How very different things are today. No matter where she travels, from her hometown of Philadelphia, Pennsylvania or the far reaches of Cuenca, Ecuador her powerful gift of healing is known. She has arrived and the world has embraced her. And from the sound of it, she does not plan to slow down anytime soon. I am grateful for her inspiration. She has been the best role-model I could imagine. I wish you safe travels Mom as you continue to amaze and to heal.

Melanie Harada

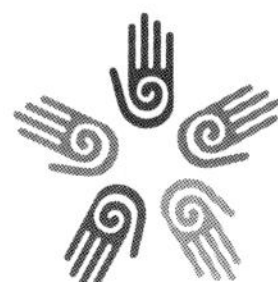

Acknowledgments

I want to acknowledge all of my friends, clients, and associates who have helped with the creation of this book. As a result of writing *Healer's Hands, Healer's Heart*, I have forged many new relationships and have had the opportunity to introduce energetic healing to my new friends.

I am deeply indebted to Ellen Reid, my Book Shepherd, who is an amazing and gifted friend. Without Ellen and her staff, *Healer's Hands, Healer's Heart* would still be an unpublished manuscript and that would be a travesty. From the start of this project, Ellen recognized the importance of this book and how it would benefit readers who are seeking alternative ways of health care. Thank you, Ellen, for keeping me on track and supporting my mission and passion.

I want to thank my assistant, Erin Bushey, who patiently acted as a very competent liaison to Ellen's staff. She provided all the necessary changes and saw to details that would have been impossible for me to manage.

And, lastly, I want to thank my lovely daughter, Melanie Harada, who thoughtfully and creatively introduced her mother to you.

SECTION I
My World as a Healer

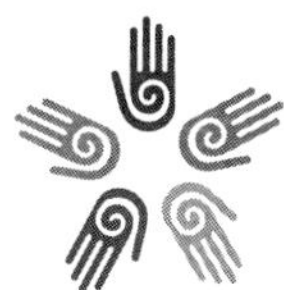

C h a p t e r   1

My Background and Frequently Asked Questions

I was originally trained as a psychotherapist, beginning my professional career in 1973. My doctorate in clinical psychology was hard won, as my dissertations on yoga and mental health were severely challenged. For many years, the political climate dictated that I describe my work in clinical terms such as "relaxation therapy," "stress reduction," and "pain management." The climate has since changed, but not fast enough.

In other cultures, the healer is well respected. However, in North America I am often met with skepticism. What many people don't realize is that this elegantly simple gift can quickly speed a healing process and at the same time complement modern medicine. The time has arrived for healers to join the growing number of alternative health care professionals.

This book addresses my personal experiences with healing in addition to its benefits as a complement to holistic health care in today's world. Yet before we begin, allow me to answer some frequently asked questions in order to share with you a little more about myself and what brought me to discover this passion.

How did you know you were a healer?

Initially, I had no idea I was a healer nor did I have any idea what healers do. However, in retrospect, I can say that I was born a healer and have always intuitively known how to take care of people. My first recollection of a healing occurred when I was sixteen years old. A friend of mine was experiencing severe pain and, as we sat together, I sensed that her pain was lessened.

Many years later, another friend of mine who had been a dancer reported back to me that after I had massaged her foot, she no longer experienced pain. In fact, she had been pain-free for two years when she reported this to me. It was then that I realized that I was a healer.

How has your Russian heritage influenced you?

All of my grandparents emigrated from Russia to America in the early 1900s. My maternal grandmother's sister was named Gittle Usherenko; her Anglicized name was Katie Share. Katie was a kind woman who used to make people feel better when they were sick. She may not have been acknowledged as a hands-on-healer during her time, but somehow people used to feel better when Katie helped them.

I was named after Katie. She died at age 41 before I was born. It is difficult to say with absolute certainty that I inherited her gift; however, upon reflection, I have always known how to help people and it was no coincidence that I was named after her.

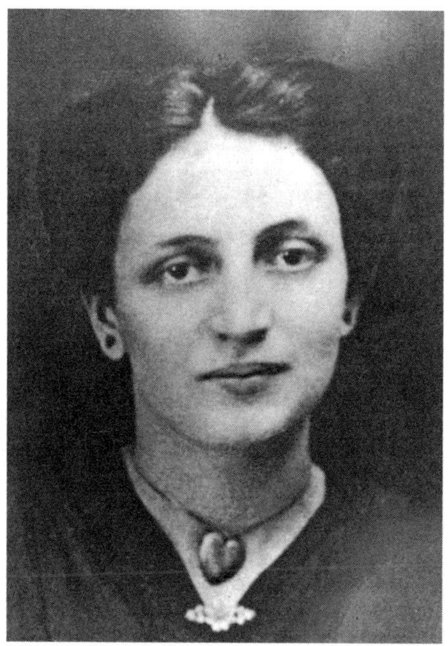

Katie Share (Gittle Usherenko)

In 1985 I felt compelled to visit Russia. I immediately felt at home. One of the most significant events during my trip occurred when I met the Russian healer, Barbara Ivanova. Barbara was a stocky, grandmotherly type who readily agreed to meet me at the hotel. I had been given her name by an American organization. She had much contact with foreigners, and since she was a linguist, we had no language difficulties.

Barbara did a hands-on-healing on a friend who accompanied me. She had my friend, Douglas, sit in a chair, and she placed her hands on his head. After about five minutes, she removed her hands from his head. We had taken a sample of Douglas's handwriting prior to the healing. His lifelong experiences with dyslexia adversely affected his writing and reading skills. After the healing, his hand-writing was more fluid and there were fewer spelling errors.

Barbara and I met many times during my stay in Russia, and I was even able to broaden my understanding of certain aspects of healing.

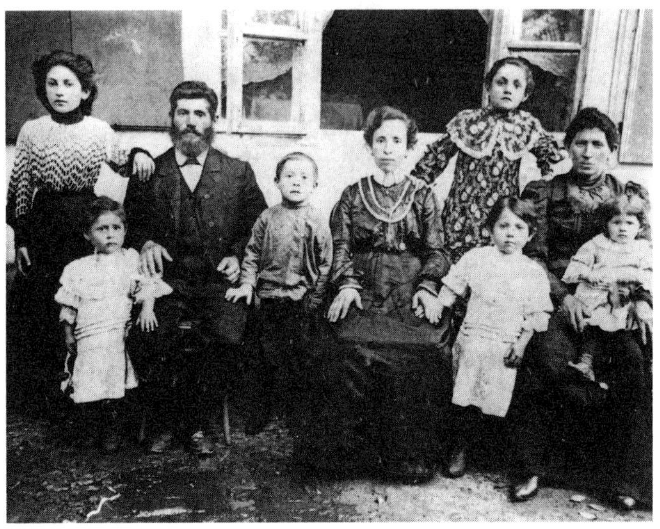

The Usherenko Family In Russia (1906)

How do you know what to do?

I work intuitively, allowing my hands to lead me. Many times, my hands will seek areas that appear to be unrelated to the complaint areas. For example, a woman with arthritis came to see me complaining of pain in her right index finger and right thumb. I began by having her sit on a chair with her back to me. There were several areas on her back that attracted me, so I placed my hands on those areas. After about ten minutes, my client broke the silence by politely reminding me about the pain in her hand. I laughed and told her that I hadn't forgotten about her pain but that I also suspected that her areas of arthritis were starting to disperse. I asked her to test her finger and thumb. Sure enough, her pain was diminished. I continued working on her back and consulted with her again. She was pain-free although I had not touched her hand.

When I work with animals, I also act spontaneously. The difference with animals is that I have to be aware of the changes that are taking place when that animal is being infused. Animals frequently need to integrate the energy during the session, and they will sometimes need to walk around, stretch, urinate, or defecate.

Where do you get your power?

First of all, it is not my power, and I prefer to think of this process as a God-given gift. I also believe that my energy fields have been enhanced by the many years that I have practiced yoga. This daily discipline is a very important part of my life. In over forty years, I only missed two months of yoga and an occasional day here and there. I realize that many individuals are interested in yoga and have practiced as diligently as I have, but my sense is that the yoga has affected my gifts in a very positive manner.

I also believe in a higher consciousness and God. My religion at birth was Jewish, and I feel that I am part of a lineage of Russian mystics. Sometimes when I do my work, I can see many women in line behind me. They are guiding and assisting me. When I am with a sick or disabled person, I frequently sense that another force is present. I revere my gift and am conscious that my mission is to use my gifts in a loving, helpful manner.

There are so many unknowns regarding my gift. Personally, I am comfortable with the knowledge that there are many of us who are healers, and in these times of global transitions, we are freer to implement our gifts. The times are rapidly changing. There is a large body of evidence that indicates that these global transitions are embracing a new consciousness, including the way people view healing.

Michael Stulberg, M.D., beautifully sums up the healing experience. He says that he is an extremely practical man and that "…whatever Gloria does, works!"

What do you do during a session?

When a client comes to my office for the first time, I request a short patient history and ask questions that are pertinent to the situation. I am most concerned with the location and nature of the complaint and the length of time the individual has been suffering. I make visual assessments during the initial interview and look for imbalances in the face. I then consider the skewness of the entire body. For instance, are the shoulders sloping symmetrically? Are the hips aligned? Is there an imbalance along the neck and head?

The interview process usually lasts fifteen minutes. In addition to assessing imbalances, I try to determine which areas of the body are compensating for injury or trauma. Nothing is in isolation; everything is connected. If the hand has been injured, chances are that the arm and shoulder have also been affected. This creates an even greater imbalance. I frequently attend to the injured area after I have made corrections elsewhere in the body. I have found that when the energy is flowing freely through the body, the affected area will be more prepared to receive the healing energy.

The intensity of my touch is light, about the same as one would use when gently touching the eyelids. I begin the session in one of two ways. If I begin by working on a client's back, he or she is seated on a chair in front of me. Often, I have the client lie down on a low massage table. Clients lie on their backs even if the complaint is in the back because it is easier for me to correct the imbalances using a frontal approach.

The session usually lasts about one hour. At the end of the session, many clients experience mild lightheadedness. This usually passes within three to five minutes. The intervention is so subtle that frequently new clients do not think that anything is happening. When they sit up and the room is spinning, they have evidence that "something has happened."

Many times new clients will feel sleepy after their initial session. My explanation for this phenomenon is that the amount of cellular activity that occurs is monumental and this intense activity causes drowsiness. In the past, clients reported that they immediately felt better after a treatment, but I really didn't have any idea why this was the case. Then one day, I was asked to visit a woman in the hospital who was being sustained intravenously. Her arms were dotted with black and blue bruises, making it difficult to find her veins. After a forty-five-minute session, the discoloration on her arms had disappeared! This was the first bit of objective evidence I had that the cellular activity was responsible for the reversal.

Is this Reiki?

The system of hands-on-healing that I have honed is different from a Reiki treatment. It is true that both systems use an energy to create change. The uniqueness of this hands-on-healing system has to do with the placement of the hands.

In this system, correcting skeletal imbalances are a key to a successful healing. The structure of the body usually reflects areas of deficit and over-energy. By energetically releasing the muscles and ligaments that are holding the body in a skewed manner, energy is able to flow more easily. As a result, deficits and areas of over-energy are corrected.

When would someone go to an energy healer?

Individuals seek the help of a healer at different stages of recovery. Some clients will see a healer before and after a surgery. The healing energy transmitted by a healer usually reduces the trauma of surgery and promotes a more rapid recovery.

Mothers with young children may consult a healer if they are determined to treat their children naturally. Others will consult a healer when several courses of antibiotics have not been effective.

There is also a group of individuals who have exhausted all possibilities in their search for optimal health. More than one client has looked at me with desperate, sad eyes and said, "You're my last hope." I used to be very disturbed by these comments. Of course, it is a huge responsibility and I am aware that I do the best I can with everyone who walks through my office door. That being said, I no longer react to individuals who believe that I am their "last hope."

The truth of the matter is that I am able to help well over 90 percent of individuals who walk through the door. Some have full resolutions in a session or two while others choose to address transformational issues that may take several months.

It is a very pleasurable experience for me when an individual is no longer in pain. Frequently, after a session, a person will make movements that prior to the session would have caused them pain; they are delighted to find that they can now function without pain.

Do you have to believe in healing for it to work?

No, one does not have to be a believer. For example, an 18 hand horse doesn't believe or disbelieve. It just works. The energy is transmitted to the horse; the horse then relaxes, and most frequently the eyelids flutter and then close. The horse is so relaxed that it becomes necessary for the horse to brace against falling. There is the evidence that energy is being transmitted.

The energy does the work. My job is to assess the imbalances and find the point of insertion. Discovering the point of insertion can amount to an intuitive roadmap. A client was having pain on the left side of her neck. I placed my hand on the right side of her neck and her left clavicle. There was no real rhyme or reason for this, but working intuitively this was a correct choice. Her pain dissipated.

Arthritic conditions respond beautifully to this system. A well-known English healer, Harry Edwards, reasoned that the heat from a healer is different from thermal heat, and the healer therefore is able to disperse the calcium carbonate associated with arthritis.

Since the energy clearly does the work, it is not necessary for a client to believe or disbelieve. It is only necessary for the client to show up.

How long do the effects of the healing last?

Once the body is in balance, the effects of the treatments can last indefinitely. Some individuals show up in my office and expect miracles. Some pain does in fact resolve after one session while some chronic conditions can take months of treatment. For example, Judy needs a tune-up every once in a while. She is quite athletic and can create an imbalance in her body from lifting weights or a demanding run. Her thirteen-year-old daughter, Linda, is athletic and has a chronic neck problem. I work on Linda occasionally, and the treatment lasts until the next trauma.

In the case of chronic fatigue syndrome, a devastating illness that can totally incapacitate even the hardiest of souls, recovery is slow and tedious and may need multiple sessions for a period of two to three months. However, a full and lasting recovery can be expected for this disorder.

Migraines can resolve in one session, or ongoing contact may be necessary. One woman in her thirties had complete resolution of her problem in just one session. Another client has occasional recurrences that are related to her menstrual cycle. When she experiences significant cramping, imbalances will appear in her face and she will get a slight headache. However, as her body becomes accustomed to a state of balance, her headaches are not as devastating as they were when she first consulted me.

One client had used a lift in his shoe for the past ten years. After our first session, he was aligned enough that he decided to remove the lift. This illustrates that the effects of the treatments have many variables. Overall, the intensity of the original complaint and the duration of the complaint are nearly always reduced. Even if there is additional trauma, one rarely goes back to square one. In very simple terms, the lasting effects of the healing depend upon the body's ability to maintain balance.

It is important to note that if a client repeatedly does the same action that is causing stress, it is not likely that the effects of treatment will last. On the other hand, if this repeated action is interrupted, the results of the healing will most likely last.

What does it feel like to do a healing?

I have many different sensations and experiences when I do a healing. At the beginning of a session, I usually feel a physical resistance to my touch. The area in which there is a physical resistance can vary from the size of my thumbnail to the surface of a limb. The physical resistance is usually very subtle and basically feels like a hard surface.

When I make my initial evaluation, I determine the areas of distress and imbalance. The light pressure that I apply activates the resistant area and allows energy to begin to move through the client. As the resistant areas soften, there is more of a balance between the left and right side of the body. For instance, frequently with a knee problem there will be an imbalance in the quadriceps. As the tone or density of the quads become more similar, knee pain can be relieved. It appears that the energy disperses the resistant areas.

As the session progresses, clients usually experience a heaviness. A 6' 9" basketball player said that during his session, this feeling of heaviness prevented him from moving. Individuals frequently feel as if they have been sedated. When I work on animals, they are also likely to respond in this manner. Horses will frequently brace their front legs. Their lower lips will quiver and they can hardly keep their eyelids open. Many horse lovers have commented that these reactions are similar to the ones they have observed after their animals have been intramuscularly sedated. As these changes occur, there is an energy that surrounds the client or animal. It is a sensation that is almost palpable. The room begins to feel thick with an energy that has a heavy yet sweet quality to it.

On occasion, I will feel a vibration moving through my finger-tips, but most often my hands do not feel as if they have a special quality to them. Sometimes my hands will feel cold to me, yet clients will still report that they feel a warmth coming from them. Clients will sometimes report that they feel as if an electrical charge is moving through their bodies. Sometimes they feel cold or numbness. In a few cases, clients will have no sensations but will still experience the benefits of the healing.

Every once in a while, I will actually experience a variation of my client's distress. The most comical of these experiences occurred when I began to notice a skin irritation on my tongue. My client had been experiencing discomfort on her tongue and before I knew what was happening, I, too, had a similar discomfort. After several glasses of water and a brisk walk around the block, I was fine. I am also likely to pick up on a client's gastrointestinal complaint. When this happens, I belch until the energy has moved the discomfort.

Does the healing drain you or make you tired?

I pace myself by choosing not to do more than four or five sessions on any given day. Since the healing energy seems to flow through me, the work does not take my energy. It is, however, extremely concentrated, and after two hours of direct contact with clients I am ready for a break. I do not go into a trance when I do the work. Sometimes, to put my client at ease, I talk about life, my children, the weather, you name it. My concentration is not affected by talking. At other times, we may both choose to be quiet. Frequently, clients will fall asleep during a session.

My office has a very soothing effect on people, so I believe that a healing energy has built up in the room where I do my work. A woman who accompanied a client to our session said that as soon as she walked in, she felt calm, relaxed, and instantly energized. While I was working on the client, this woman felt the increase in energy throughout the room, and she was seated about five feet away from the treatment table.

When I work with some clients, I become energized. The energetic communion becomes profound and I, in fact, feel infused with energy. Sometimes when I am this way, I will feel elated and tired at the same time. I have an experience that is similar to the ones my clients experience when there is intense and prolific cellular activity.

How did you learn to do long-distance healing?

My first experience with long-distance healing was in Moscow with Barbara Ivanova. We sat across from each other, and Barbara said, "Look at me now." I gazed into her eyes, and I was transfixed. She held me in this manner for approximately sixty seconds. Then she said, "OK." It was a strange sensation to be mesmerized in this manner.

Barbara was best known for her telephone healing, and she was kind enough to show me what she does during her long-distance work. I called Barbara at her home, and she demonstrated the telephone healing. She asked me to place the phone to my left ear while she held the phone to her right ear. As her energy was transferred, Barbara initiated the healing. It was very subtle. I felt a transmission and movement of energy throughout my body.

When I returned to the States, I began to dabble with long-distance healing. Barbara's influence gave me the impetus to develop another technique that is quite different yet very effective.

When I do long-distance healing, I get an impression about the distresses in the body and on paper draw very crude impressions of the areas of distress. I mark these areas with X's and hang a pendulum over the areas. The pendulum is an object that is well weighted and has the ability to pick up an energy and vibrate with that energy,. This is a process called radionics. The pendulum rotates counterclockwise while the aura clears. As the healing energy enters the body, the rotation moves to a clockwise rotation. Clients will usually begin to feel better within one to five minutes, perhaps longer if they are farther away.

Very interesting successes with long-distance healing have occurred since I started practicing this technique. I consider it a very important part of my practice. (I discuss my long-distance healing system and the pendulum more in Chapter 8: Healing for Beginners.)

Can anybody heal?

This is a very difficult question for me, and I would tend to believe that the answer is "yes." Anybody can heal, but not everyone is a healer. My definition of healing has to do with a transmission of a subtle energy. My older daughter, who is a relatively new mother, stated, "No one can heal my child the way I can. When I hold my son and touch him when he is hurt, no one can come close to giving him what I give him." I believe my daughter is correct, and yet certain conditions require additional energy.

My responsibility to my clients is very compelling. For instance, I feel that once I have connected with someone, I am connected and available indefinitely. Yet, I have clear limits. When I was contacted by an intoxicated, disturbed client, I recommended that he call a counselor or go to the emergency room. I do not deal with anyone who is using recreational drugs, as it is not good for me to be around that energy, and I do not knowingly expose myself to a client who is emitting a toxic energy that could be transferred to me.

Out of deference to my clients, I wash my hands before and after each session. I immediately wash to rid my hands of any needless energy that I may have collected. In Durango, Mexico, I worked on many poverty-stricken individuals and was in several primitive settings. One of these places was a barn where I had worked on a woman who had open sores. There was no running water, but there was lots of tequila; I cleansed my hands with very hardy tequila. I learned my lesson with that experience, so now I usually take a small bottle of rubbing alcohol with me if I am going into an underdeveloped area.

As a healer, I am always conscious that I am merely a vehicle. I take no credit for the actual healing. The energy flows through me, making me the conduit. I do not like the word "power" in connection with healing but rather the word "gifted." There's a reverence and detachment connected to "gifted." Healing is not about an ego trip.

Individuals who have a keen interest in energy work usually have a propensity for healing. It is not difficult to learn to bring energy to your hands. Many individuals are able to do this without instruction. When a child is hurt and the parent instinctively rubs the area that has been injured, an energy is transferred to the child. However, in less obvious situations, one needs to learn about hand placement for the most effective outcome. The hands are not usually placed on the distressed area. For instance, a sore throat can be most effectively treated by placing hands on the back of the neck. Intuitively, one needs to find the area on the neck that corresponds to the sore throat.

In the case of a knee injury, the inside of the thigh is frequently disturbed. If the practitioner only touched the knee, it is unlikely that a full resolution would occur.

People often wonder, "How much can you teach?" As I have said, it is not difficult to bring energy to the hands; the difficult task is to train individuals to have increased intuition about the most effective hand placements.

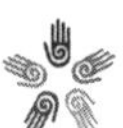

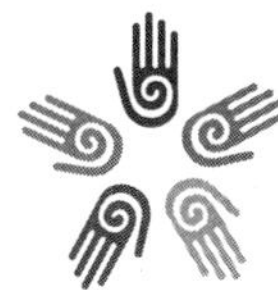

Dramatic Healings
Of Everyday People

An Interview with Patti

Patti is a singer and composer. She is the mother of three children and has called on me many times to help with her family's various complaints. I first met Patti and her mother at a yoga class.

Patti: Having grown up in Nebraska, we just weren't taught to believe in the kinds of things you do. My mother was visiting and, jokingly, you volunteered to give my mother a "strange California experience." You asked mother if she had any aches or pains. I don't remember her exact words, but she basically said that everything was fine. I reminded my mom of her hip injury. Seven or eight years before, she had hurt her hip helping me move some boxes, and her hip has hurt her ever since. I can't remember where you touched my mother. You laid your hands somewhere on her, and the pain got better. My mother's injury occurred when I was in my twenties; she has since passed, but never in all of her years had that hip problem return.

Dr. Kaye: You and I did a few sessions together after that. You have a curvature in your spine that caused you pain.

Patti: I never got a good night's sleep, always having to shift from one side to the other because of the back pain. It got to the point where I was very uncomfortable driving the car. I then came to see you. If I had to look to my side while doing parallel parking, I was very uncomfortable. I had been to chiropractors in Las Vegas and California. They took X-rays, and it was the second chiropractor who told me I needed a lift in one shoe. I had the lift built into all my shoes. It helped somewhat, but I still was uncomfortable. After I visited you, you said, "I don't think you need those lifts in your shoes." I took out the lift, and my pain disappeared.

Dr. Kaye: My next recollection of associating with your family was coming to your house and seeing your young son, Ryan. He was having a problem with his asthma. I remember he was looking for my wand. He wanted to know where the fairy godmother's "wand" and sparkles were.

Patti: You were very helpful to Ryan. His congestion and stuffiness cleared up. I remember you asking, "Is it better?" And he'd say, "Well, I can breathe on this side now." Then, you did the other sinus points, and it was instant relief for him.

I'd just like to say one other thing that happened with Ryan. I used to diagnose learning disabilities, and I've always felt that Ryan had a learning disability. After one of the times you worked with him, he was waiting for me to complete my session and started to do his homework. He copied his words while he was sitting and waiting, and it was done perfectly with no reversals. He'd had problems with that before. He might have been quite young at the time, maybe five or six. I asked you about it, and you said very often it does help with that kind of thing. I thought that was very interesting.

Dr. Kaye: When Brittany was about twenty months old, she had projectile vomiting. She was getting dehydrated. That was kind of scary.

Patti: The doctors felt that the vomiting came from a malfunction that would eventually correct. Anyway, you did help with that. Her whole meal or whatever she nursed would be totally gone. It went on all day long, all the time. The doctors just said that some things just do not close off until a certain age. You worked on her, and that condition improved dramatically.

Dr. Kaye: She had the flu and eczema.

Patti: Not at the same time, but she did have the flu once, and she couldn't even keep her water down. She was so sick, and I remember she lost a few pounds. She didn't even look like my little girl anymore, and honestly, I was afraid she might die. She was throwing up blood. Her little tummy had nothing left in it, and after she visited you, she did improve. The eczema was a different story. She had this terrible rash all over her. I took her to see you, but first, I took her to see the pediatrician. He asked if I changed laundry detergents. You know, all the things to try and figure out what on earth was causing her problem. I don't know if she was on solid foods yet, but something was causing this rash all over her body. It wouldn't go away. She had it for quite some time when I brought her to see you. You made a paste with a homeopathic remedy and applied it in a circular area on her tummy and said, "Check this and if this works; go to the health food store for ferrous phosphate. Make a paste, and put it on her." I looked later that day where you had put this circle; there was no rash where the circle was. I thought we found the solution. I went to the health food store, got the ferrous phosphate, made the muddy paste, and coated her entire body with it. It didn't do a thing. I then realized that it was Gloria. Where Gloria had put the ferrous phosphate, the rash had completely cleared up.

Dr. Kaye: That was quite an experience for me, too. Patti's been my teacher helping me see the potentials of this healing. After that, Ryan fell off his bike.

Patti: Oh yes. My son had a bike accident where his front wheel fell off, and he landed on his head. He had a concussion. You worked on him after that incident. He had been hospitalized and had a CAT scan. I was afraid he was going to lose his front tooth. It was discolored, so I took him to the children's dentist. They gave him the ice test, and he had no feeling in that tooth. They were going to see about doing some surgery on the tooth. He said I could wait a few months, but if it was his child, he wouldn't. I decided to let you take a look at him. You didn't say for sure you could help, but you worked on him. His tooth, till this day, is fine. It's perfectly colored. He has had no trouble with that tooth so far. I really feel like you saved his tooth…and he did not have to go through the root canal. I'm amazed.

Dr. Kaye: Let's see, what else did we do? Recently, we…

Patti: You worked on Gary's hand.

Dr. Kaye: Gary's still a little bit of a skeptic.

Patti: My husband is an avid golfer. He loves golf! At one time, he was considering becoming a professional golfer. He's played in the U.S. Open. His hand started hurting him so badly that he couldn't play golf anymore. He'd come in after a hole or two because he was in such pain. He was convinced he had arthritis or cancer. He's a little bit of a hypochondriac. You worked on his hand, and after that first time he's back golfing. I think you worked on him a couple times after that. He doesn't complain anymore.

Dr. Kaye: Thank you very much.

Pele's Magical Encounter

Hawaii has always been a magical place for me. I was on my way back from Tripler Army Medical Center in Honolulu, where I had lectured on alternative healing methods for AIDS patients. I found myself in one of those magical situations that should be relegated to true romance novels. Because of my red hair, more than one believer has questioned whether I am Pele (with deepest respect). I always smile and deny the possibility. For those of you who are not familiar with the legend, Pele is the Hawaiian volcano goddess of fire who has red hair and can appear as a very young, beautiful woman or as an old crone.

The man seated next to me on the small commuter plane looked at me questioningly. Was I or was I not Madame Pele? He was a stuntman returning to his home in Kona, and I was on my way to visit a friend. We chatted briefly on the short commuter trip, and I told him that I had just lectured at Tripler Army Medical Center. He was interested and asked me many questions about my work. When I told him that I specialized in pain management, his face brightened.

He began to tell me his story. He had an old injury that he sustained while doing a movie stunt. His shoulder constantly throbbed, and he had tried everything in an attempt to alleviate the pain. I asked him if he wanted me to try to help him; he jumped at the offer. He wanted to know when we would be able to do this, and I told him that if he didn't have any problem with my working on him during the flight then I was game for a spontaneous healing.

I placed my hands on his right shoulder and began to infuse him with energy. He closed his eyes and melted into the experience. Within a short time, I felt as if the corrections were complete. I asked him to raise his arm. He was able to do so without any discomfort. He was astonished. He asked me endless questions, but before we knew it our commuter ride had ended. We exchanged telephone numbers, and although we had no further communication there is a special place in my heart for the stuntman who wondered who he sat next to that day.

The Big Turnaround

I love New York and a New York sense of humor and wit. David was a very young seventy-five-year-old transplant from NYC. He definitely had questions about me and what I was doing. He had been to many practitioners seeking relief from the pain he experienced in his feet. He checked out New York's finest physicians and also consulted nontraditional East Coast practitioners. He consulted traditional and nontraditional practitioners on the West coast as well before deciding to call me. He heard about my work through a friend who had a monkey that I had worked on. David looked at me and said, "If you can heal a monkey, maybe you can heal me." I looked at him and said, "Maybe."

I was taking care of elderly people when I met David. My office was in my care home. I know he was puzzled while he followed me back to the office. It had a sophisticated turn-of-the-century look to it with lace, dried flowers, and soft lighting.

David looked around the office and asked where I kept my potions and dried bones. I laughed and told him that I kept the bones in the closet and my secret potions in a wall safe. He looked at me and laughed. The ice was broken.

I assured David that my massage table was just an ordinary one without any magical charms or imbedded crystals. I did tell him, however, that the chair in which I was sitting was my great-Aunt Katie's and that it was special for me. David was becoming less skeptical. I think he also liked my wit.

Having made my assessment of David's physical complaints, I immediately found the imbalances that were contributing to his problems. He had a misalignment in his neck and hips, which caused him to place undue stress on his feet.

Working on him while he was in a sitting position, his neck softened. He was pleased with that improvement. I then had him lie down on the massage table. He was grinning from ear to ear as his imagination provided him with many pleasant images. As we got to know each other better, he shared some of his very funny thoughts. He had me laughing through most of the sessions.

After just a few sessions, David's original complaints resolved. David wrote a support letter. I present it to you in its entirety so you can get the flavor of this wonderful man:

> *I am not a cynic, but I am a skeptic. Especially when it comes to Southern California HEALERS.*
>
> *I am a skeptic no longer!*

Fifteen or more years ago, an eminent podiatrist diagnosed the pains in my feet while jogging to be from arthritis. I tried every method I could find to reduce the pain—from massage to hypnosis, from Feldenkrais to acupuncture to psychology, etc.—all to no avail, except Feldenkrais, which reduced the pain some.

I have just had two sessions with healer/Doctor Gloria Kaye. After the first one, my pain was relieved by half. And three days later, after the second, the pain has disappeared COMPLETELY!

And while she was treating me she also used her methodology to free my neck movement, which was restricted for at least forty (40) years due to calcium deposits revealed by X-rays. Restricted no longer, I now can move my neck freely in any direction!

Doctor Kaye does more than HEAL! She performs MIRACLES!!

As you can see, David became a big fan of mine. He referred several family members, and I was embraced by the whole family.

Healing and Rejuvenation

Another relocated New Yorker who vastly impressed me was a seventy-nine-year-old retired CEO. He and his wife lived on a small ranch in Santa Maria, California. Their 150-year-old house was quite amazing and restored in such a manner that you felt as if you were visiting folks from yesteryear.

Lester had arthritis in his hands and feet. He was in constant pain and tried everything to restore his mobility and get some relief from this chronic situation. Lester and his wife, Adrienne, heard about me through some friends, and in those days I was making regular house calls.

I explained how the heat from a healer helps to disperse most of the calcium carbonate associated with arthritis, as well as the fact that most people feel better after a treatment. I held Lester's hand. He looked at me, smiled and said, "I think I'm going to like this!" I worked on both of Lester's hands, and then I asked if there were somewhere that I could work where he could lie down. We decided to go into the guest bedroom where there were two twin beds. Adrienne followed us, and we decided that the bed on the right would be most suitable as it allowed me to work on Lester from his right side. Lester stretched out on the bed and immediately became relaxed.

The scene was a very peaceful one. Lester was lying on one bed with a delighted grin on his face. Adrienne was lying on the other bed and she too was looking serene. The dogs had joined us. They were also calm. I closed my eyes and continued to work on Lester. It was an idyllic setting. As I felt the peaceful energy permeating the room, I also became conscious of Lester's very regular breathing. When I took a closer look I realized that he was sleeping. I was somewhat disconcerted when I heard regular breathing coming from the other side of the room. I knew this couldn't be an echo, but it certainly was strange.

I followed the sound and behind a large club chair, two lightly snoring mongrels were sound asleep. I just shook my head and smiled at the potency of the energy. I went back to my chair by the side of the bed and was bothered by yet another series of regular breathing sounds. Perhaps there was an echo after all!

No, it was Adrienne. She was sound asleep in the other bed. Then I cleared my throat and made noises to rouse this crew. They were all very surprised by the fact that they all fell asleep. Lester laughed and asked if I could come live with them. His hands felt better, and he walked more fluidly. We decided to meet again the following week.

The next session immediately duplicated the previous one. Within five minutes Lester, Adrienne, and the two dogs were out cold. This was getting to be a lonely experience. I decided to close my eyes and relax along with them. I never have fallen asleep during a session, so I felt confident that I would remain awake. As I was relaxing, however, I heard some stirring and opened my eyes. It was Lester. Although he was sound asleep, he began to make some decidedly sensual body movements. They were so sensual that I wondered what this man was like thirty years ago. His delicate, arthritic hands massaged the entire front of his body as he suggestively moved his hips. I felt extremely awkward. I did not want to wake him and at the same time I would have been a bit of a voyeur if I continued to watch the show. My solution to this dilemma was to move to the end of the bed. I turned my back on this seductive scene and worked on Lester's feet. It seemed like a more private way to handle the situation. I have to admit that I was tempted to peek but propriety prevailed, and Lester didn't have me as an audience.

When the work was complete I made more disturbing, throat-clearing noises, and within minutes the group was conscious. Immediately, Lester popped up and his first words were, "Did I hurt you?" I answered, "No" and he said, "Thank God." He said that he had a dream but he couldn't possibly tell me about it. I coaxed him and he told me that he had an unusual dream. He dreamed that his left leg had an erection. He said his leg felt warm, hard, and very alive. With a big grin on his face, he asked me if I could do the same thing to his right leg! We were all hysterical with laughter. I told him that I would see what I could do.

The next week when I returned, Lester asked, "What did you do to me? I have had spontaneous erections for the last week. Do you want to see?" I congratulated him and told him that it would not be necessary to see his newfound apparatus. He was a little disappointed.

The banter went on and on including Lester's suggestion that he and I start a little clinic for some of his friends. Needless to say, Lester was feeling no pain and was a happy camper.

Getting Back on Your Feet

My beautiful Australian friend, Margo, called me at home. She apologized for calling me at home, but she was in intense pain and had not slept for the past two nights. She had a badly sprained foot and was unable to put any weight on it. She asked if I could possibly come over to her apartment and do a healing on the foot.

It was after 8 p.m., and because of my commitment to lead a balanced life, I usually do not do healings in the evenings. I learned early that many healers had injured themselves from overwork and exhaustion. However, Margo would not have called unless there was a very serious situation. She had a sleep disorder and this, compounded with her injury, was more than she could tolerate. When I arrived at her apartment, she was nestled on the sofa in a fetal-like position. The dark circles under her eyes gave her an even more haunted look. Her suffering was obvious.

My heart went out to her. I began the work and as usual, I did not begin on the area of distress. Her back was affected by the trauma to her foot. I began working on her shoulders and slowly moved to her back. She released a sigh and closed her eyes. The pain in her back was starting to lift. I worked on her head to ease her emotions. You could almost see the thoughts that were going on in her head. Her brow was crevassed like a rock climber's fantasy. After a few minutes of work on her cranium, this stubborn Aussie started to let go.

I was able to move to her knee and calf to infuse these areas with energy. Her leg was getting very warm. I finally placed my hand on her foot, and it began to ease the pain. I held my hand on her foot for several minutes. When the area felt normal to my touch, I removed my hand and asked Margo how she was feeling. She said that she was much better, and she tried to stand.

She was able to put her full weight on the foot but did not trust that she could walk on the foot. I told her it would be all right, and I stood by her side. She walked tentatively and then realized that she actually walked normally on the foot.

She looked at me and said, "I don't believe this. How did you do that?" Margo got quite excited and actually started to hop on her foot. I stopped her from doing that right away. I didn't want to push a good thing.

Margo recovered fully that night. I suggested that she wear supported shoes for the next forty-eight hours. Margo kindly wrote the following letter of endorsement:

Last week, after badly spraining my ankle, I was immobilized with severe pain and a regimen of bed rest, ice packs and aspirin.

I was naturally upset and frustrated because in my past experience, injuries of this kind are usually extremely debilitating. Healing and full recovery usually take weeks and often months to be effective.

Gloria placed her hands on my ankle for about forty-five minutes in total, during which I experienced some "warming" sensations and several sharp and painful pulsations along my lower leg.

At the end of the treatment I was asked to stand with my weight naturally and evenly distributed, and then to walk.

I was astonished and delighted when I found that I could do both easily and without pain.

It was an extraordinary experience, and the next day, after being advised only to wear shoes with adequate support, I was walking freely and naturally! And most importantly, pain-free.

The Finger: A Miraculous Sight

I met Laurel through her daughter, Janet. Laurel had lived through World War II, and there was a certain reluctance and skepticism about her that I have seen among individuals who have experienced unbearable trauma. She is a beautiful woman and had been a teacher. She was writing her memoirs and at eighty-one had just learned how to use a personal computer. Laurel had a no-nonsense spirit of adventure about her.

Janet was paying Laurel a weekend visit and decided to contact me while she was in the area. Janet had chronic pain in her feet and when she called me, she was at her wit's end. I saw Janet at Laurel's apartment, so Laurel was able to watch me work. At the end of our hour, Janet was no longer in pain. She had a number of imbalances that actually resolved within our first session. Both Janet and Laurel were impressed and so Laurel later contacted me. She had a bone spur that she wanted me to reduce. I saw her several times, and her pain was diminished. She wasn't convinced that the bone spur was resolving, and I certainly wasn't going to argue with her.

Laurel called to cancel an appointment because she had injured her finger. I encouraged her to keep the appointment with me so that I could help her with her finger as well as the bone spur. Being the stoic person that she is, she did not immediately tell me the details of her accident. Eventually, she told me that she had closed a car door on her finger. She told the story calmly. She and her daughter-in-law had been shopping, and when Laurel got in the car she slammed the door on her finger and actually lost part of her finger on the door. They went to Laurel's apartment to call the family doctor. He told them to go to the emergency room, where Laurel had her finger X-rayed. There were no breaks, but a hand specialist was consulted. He thought that a skin graft might be needed, but he wanted to give it a few days before any decisions were made.

When I arrived at Laurel's apartment, the door had been left open for me. Laurel was in her bedroom with her bandaged finger. She looked a little pale. I asked her to rest in her bed while I worked on her.

I began to run energy through her body and worked on the shoulder and forearm of her injured hand. She relaxed and I worked my way along her hand, eventually running energy directly to her finger. As I continued to do this, it appeared as if the skin underneath the injury was puffing up. It was hard to believe, but before our eyes we could see the wound healing. As we both watched in disbelief, the affected area started to reduce in size. The area was not only healing from underneath, it also was shrinking. I have witnessed this phenomenon several times, and each time I am totally in awe of the process.

Laurel was no longer a skeptic. She and I were both wide-eyed and reverent. She commented:

"My finger healed in four weeks. The doctor said it would take two months. It was amazing!"

A Near Tragedy

On a beautiful Saturday morning in Santa Barbara, Paula and I decided to hike the Figueroa Mountain trail. It is a fairly easy hike. We first drove through the Santa Ynez Valley before we came to the turn-off for Figueroa Mountain. The thirteen-mile drive to the trailhead was very pleasant. Grazing cattle and ranch houses tucked away in the rolling hills made the drive very sweet. The posted sign "NO SERVICES FOR THE NEXT 22 MILES" lingered in my mind.

After several miles, Paula and I decided to park the car and hike up the paved road. The sun was brilliant; there were a few lazy clouds hovering. I looked up and around at this magnificent vista, and out of the corner of my eye I saw two figures hang-gliding. They blended with the circling turkey vultures that were also catching the air currents. I felt slightly overwhelmed by the beauty surrounding us.

Paula and I were making our uphill ascent and feeling the newness of the hike. As much as I have hiked around these beautiful mountains, I always feel a little disconnected with the mind-body experience until I actually get into the rhythm of the hike. Slowly, my consciousness was shifting and my movements were becoming fluid. Again out of the corner of my eye, I glimpsed at the two figures gliding on the wind currents. They looked more like winged creatures than human figures. They appeared to be starting their descent and slowly maneuvered the gliders. Before we knew it, the first figure landed in a cow pasture about 500 feet from us. The male figure began gathering up his extensive paraphernalia. We looked for the second figure, and a beautiful young woman appeared to be sitting on an air current. She came down so gently with her legs extended in front of her. She looked as if she could have been sitting on a cloud.

To our horror, her extended legs clipped the top of a scruffy oak tree; she lost control and landed head first about twenty feet from the tree. For what seemed the longest fifteen seconds of my life, there was a stillness and quietude that I had never experienced before. I knew that I was running to this soundless creature, but my movements were automatic, coming from somewhere deep within me. By the time I arrived, this nineteen-year-old girl had regained consciousness and was in excruciating pain. She was screaming. Her shoulder was badly injured, and she was scared. She called for her friend who, by this time, had extricated himself from his harness. He came running, eyes wide with disbelief. This horror was reserved for the movies or the eleven o'clock news. He kept saying, "Karla, Karla, what can I do? What happened?"

By this time I was trying my best to begin the work. It was very important to remain calm, or I would not be able to create the atmosphere to attend to Karla. I touched her head and talked softly to her. She wanted her friend to remove her harness, but I insisted that she not move or be moved. I was wearing a cotton vest, which I took off, and by just barely adjusting her head I was able to slip the vest under her face. Having landed head first and face down, she was covered with debris and abrasions. She seemed to appreciate the slight protection for her face. I continued to talk softly to her, and in spite of everything, she quieted down.

We were soon joined by other hikers who had seen the accident. I immediately asked someone to get help. Since we were in a rather isolated area, this was a particularly difficult situation. Two hikers raced to their car and drove to the nearest phone to call for help. Time seemed to stand still.

Volunteers joined me. One man started to tell Karla about his experiences in Vietnam and what it was like when he broke his leg. A man who looked like a Native American sat by my side in prayer. Mark, the other glider, busied himself with the equipment, and as long as Karla stayed focused on her breathing and relaxing, she refrained from screaming out. People were milling around like chaotic ants. After what seemed like an interminable time, a fire truck arrived complete with a hook and ladder. The hikers who had called for help approached the first ranch that they saw, and it happened to be Michael Jackson's. The fire truck that was on the scene was Michael Jackson's private vehicle, and he kindly sent it along to assist us. The trained firefighters lent some assistance while we waited for the paramedics and an ambulance.

With the arrival of the firefighters, the entire scene changed. The energy became more frenetic and Karla was screaming again. There was tremendous agitation in the air. There was no way to explain my presence or that of my prayerful friend. We looked at each other and slowly withdrew now that the "professionals" had arrived. The shift in energy was dramatic.

We stood back and watched this gruesome scene. Would there ever be a day when there would be a place for healers? I stayed until Karla was put in the ambulance. When she was removed, it felt as if there were a large empty hole in the space she had occupied. Because of the intensity of the experience, I needed to rescue my vest and bury it along with the sadness of the scene. Paula and I hiked a bit farther until I found my spot. I buried my vest under a fallen log along with my feelings of impotence and being out of sync with this century.

Diminishing Physical and Emotional Ailments

The skeptics keep me on my toes and make it doubly important for me to stay out of the way of the ego. Jim was a certain sort of skeptic that posed an immense challenge. He was a former businessman, psychotherapist, and manager of a successful New Age center that offered alternative health interventions including acupuncture, healing, yoga, and holistic medicine. Jim had seen it all and was well connected with the alternative health community, but nevertheless he identified himself as a skeptic.

Jim wanted to experience one of my sessions. I was immediately drawn to a lipoma on the left side of his neck. This large, fatty cyst was about the size of an orange. As we proceeded with the session, he commented on, as he put it, the metaphysics of the situation. After all, if the healings dispersed his lipoma then he would have absolute proof that something occurred.

I busied myself with the healing and detached myself from Jim's agenda. I had Jim sit in a chair, and I began working on his upper body. He told me about some of his other complaints, which included mid-back pain and digestive troubles. We chatted about my aspirations and his plans for the center. I was impressed with Jim's sincerity and his adventure with the center.

After a short time, I refocused on the cyst and found that it was starting to soften. The diameter of the cyst had not changed, but as so frequently happens the quality of the affected area changed. Jim was starting to look relaxed. His entire body was less rigid, and I was then attracted to the upper portion of his skull. It was very resistant, perhaps reflecting Jim's "hardheadedness." Many individuals who are thoughtful and cerebral frequently have little elasticity or movement of the flesh covering the skull. In addition, the structural imbalances in the skull were fairly pronounced, which was also of interest to me. It appeared that there was an over-energy on the right side of Jim's skull. By infusing the right side, the energy was forced to shift to the left, creating a more balanced situation.

When I felt the need to bring the energy to Jim's feet, I assisted him to the sofa. He was a little lightheaded. It was a simple task to bring the energy down to his feet. Within minutes, Jim was breathing regularly and appeared to be asleep. When the session was complete, he awoke gently. He was feeling relaxed, and his color had changed significantly. We scheduled another appointment.

When I saw Jim five days later, his cyst had considerably reduced. I spent thirty minutes infusing the area, and at the end of our second session, the cyst had reduced between 65 and 75 percent. Jim was becoming less of a skeptic. He could now feel the change. He wanted me to meet his girlfriend, so we scheduled an appointment for the two of them.

One week later, I returned for our third and final treatment. Jim introduced me to Sue. We shook hands, looked into each other's eyes, and acknowledged our knowingness of each other. Sue excitedly showed me a tracing of the cyst she had made immediately after the second session. She had placed a piece of paper right on Jim's neck and drew a pencil line around the cyst. She proudly showed me how it had reduced in size since her tracing. We were all very encouraged.

When I began the session, I had Jim sit in a chair. Sue joined us and also sat in a chair. As soon as I began with Jim, Sue had an intense reaction. Her lower extremities trembled and then the trembling shifted to her head and torso. I had seen this reaction before, and I wasn't too concerned, except for the fact that it had the potential of interrupting my session with Jim. I did eventually stop working on Jim after a few minutes. I went over to Sue and placed my hand about an inch from the top of her head in order to pull the energy in her body upward. She immediately stopped trembling and began to have a look of serenity and calm.

By this time the energy among the three of us was very intense. It was almost as if we were all suspended in a vortex. Later, Jim described his state as a meditative one in which he called on many spiritual masters to help with the healing. Jim's body was softening and the cyst was reducing. Just before I had him lie down to complete the session, the quality of the cyst had completely changed. There was no core to the cyst. What remained of the cyst was totally soft.

I assisted Jim to the daybed. He was very lightheaded at this time. I worked on drawing the energy down to his feet. The one area that remained resistant was the crook of Jim's big left toe. This made perfect sense to me because the cyst was on his left side. I asked Jim to imagine that he was warming my fingertips as I held his toe, and within minutes the resistant spot had softened. I knew that the softening of this area would put the final touches on Jim's lipoma. Jim was resting very deeply, and I asked him to continue to rest. I washed my hands, took a deep breath, thanked God, and went over to work with Sue.

After her initial trembling, Sue had remained motionless throughout the time that I was working on Jim. When I approached her, I disturbed her meditation.

She said the calm that had come over her was very significant. Her experience was a centering one. My intuition about Sue was that we needed to move the energy throughout her body. Her physical complaints focused on uterine fibroids. She felt that the formation of the fibroids ten years ago was somehow connected to a psychological trauma.

As we walked to her bedroom to complete the session, she staggered down the hallway. The energy had made her knees weak. She chose to use the walls for support rather than for me to assist her.

As she rested on the floor of her bedroom, her imbalances became obvious. Her head cocked to the left. Her left foot was more upright than her right foot, indicating more imbalances in the hip and pelvic regions. I began by using a gentle pressure on her hipbones. The downward pressure immediately gave her a release of pressure in her lower back. She softened as her left foot also relaxed. I was then attracted to her right hand and found some resistant points there. As I worked on her hand, I sensed an image of a dark figure near her.

I asked her if she wanted to do a past life regression as a means to get to the source of her fibroids. She agreed. I asked her if she would go back to a time in history when she was assaulted. Her body stiffened and, in my mind's eye, I could see this dark figure. I wondered how long her body would remain in a stiffened state and if it would be necessary to help her out of her trance. She angrily relived a very significant past life experience of horror and humiliation. Her vagina had been penetrated by a phallic-like object, and her head had been pinned to one side. She felt as if a ritual was being performed, but she couldn't identify the ritual. The episode may have lasted five minutes. It ended as suddenly as it began.

I continued working on the imbalances and was immediately struck by the fact that Sue's head was no longer skewed to the left. I took a second look and it was true. Her head was in a normal position. She appeared to be very aligned. The work was nearly complete, and Sue rested.

When we discussed the regression, Sue also added that no one has ever been able to touch her neck on the left side, and that she always pulled away from Jim if he tried to be affectionate on the left side of her neck. I wondered if this would still be true.

We walked back into the living room, where Jim was waiting for us. We told him about the regression, and I asked him if he would try kissing Sue on her neck. As they embraced, Sue didn't flinch. The sweetness of the moment brought tears to my eyes.

An Interview with Mary

Mary was decidedly sad and overwhelmed as the mother of a lovely little girl who was severely impaired neurologically. Mary had been through the ringer trying to find help for her child, Jane. When we met, I was faced with a somewhat skeptical parent.

Mary: To give you an overview of what my situation is, I need to go back in history to five years ago. I am the parent of a little girl who at eighteen months was a normal, healthy child. Everything was in place and intact in terms of developmental milestones. Then my child received an eighteen-month immunization shot. (There are five in total.) The day after she received her immunization—actually within twelve hours—I noticed that something was up.

Initially, I saw a loss of motor control and some shaking as if she were cold. It became progressively worse. Within five days, she had deteriorated from a healthy eighteen-month-old child—running, speaking, and talking—to a child who completely lost her ability to walk. In fact, there was nothing left on the developmental scale that she could do. She had lost eye control; she had lost everything that could be lost within five days. We watched it disappear.

Dr. Kaye: What was happening to you as this was happening to your daughter?

Mary: I was devastated. To say that my heart was breaking doesn't even describe what was going on. I wanted to die. I wanted to know what was going on so that I could stop it. I had tremendous feelings of disempowerment and loss of control. I wanted to die.

Dr. Kaye: How long were you and Jane suffering before we met?

Mary: There was a period of time, perhaps three years, in which there was a very slight improvement. Her eyes were jumping and circling like cartoon eyes. Because she was unable to focus, she was unable to eat, and she was throwing up all of the time. Her inability to control her motor skills meant that she couldn't stand. She had lots of falls and lots of stitches. For those three years, that was her life. She did crawl somewhat. She drag-crawled for a long time, and then she was up on all fours again. She made some attempt to go back through the developmental milestones.

Dr. Kaye: When you first brought Jane to me, I was impressed with her spirit. Here was a child who would not give up. She would attempt to take a step, fall, and try again. As I recall, at our first session she wanted to play with the water in the sink. We managed to busy her. She was on a chair, playing with the water and some toys. I began working on her spine. I remember the strong attraction I had to her spine, even though she had all of these other complaints. Sometimes it is difficult for me to actually believe that something is going on. However, I knew something was going on. I just didn't know how it would manifest. We finished that session; she was very cooperative. Did you see an immediate change after that?

Mary: I saw that within six weeks, she was walking. You were seeing her once or twice a week. She went from a child who was falling all of the time and crawling all of the time to walking.

Dr. Kaye: How old was she at the time?

Mary: She was four and a half. I have been exposed to many questionable services. A lot of claims are built on people's hopes and dreams and frailties. People will profess that they can accomplish what they cannot. So I am a great source of credibility for you and your work. I didn't believe that anything was going to happen. I saw people pray and lay amulets on her and nothing happened. I don't know if I ever mentioned this to you because I was so overwhelmed with even talking about it.

Several times when you worked with her, you just inadvertently touched me and your hands were very hot. It created some sort of cognitive dissonance in me because what I see happening, what my eyes are telling me, and what people are reporting to me is different from my expectations and beliefs. It took a while for it to catch up, but I do know about molecular reorganization and miracles occurring. I did not know what to call this. I do not know what name to give it. What I do know is that something very significant and profound happened. My little girl was walking in about six weeks. This was a child that we were told to institutionalize. There was no hope. "Forget about it; have another child." The combination of her spirit, and you know the fighter she is, and our holding out for nothing less than a miracle got us the results we were seeking. It always happens that someone appears who is supposed to—a teacher, a guide. Then you were there. We had lost all hope. Not only did you give us back our hope; her improvement was beyond our wildest dreams.

Dr. Kaye: The last time we spoke, you were telling me that she was doing two ballet classes.

Mary: She does two ballet classes a week. She does a dance class, and she does another activities class. People continually look at her and comment that they cannot believe that she is the same child. For the last year and a half, she has attended a regular school. Her speech has dramatically improved. Since the time you started working with her, all of these things have changed. To look at her, she looks like a regular little kid, running around, getting into trouble.

What is significant to me is that I was always her sort of human translator, and now people are starting to understand her. She can make conversations with people about various things, and I hear that they are making appropriate statements back to her such as, "That was an interesting book you were telling me about." So, I know that they are not humoring her. They are actually having conversations with her. It is wonderful also now that she can be understood by her peers.

Dr. Kaye: I was attracted to working on the area of her throat the last time that we met, and so it is interesting to hear about these changes.

Mary: She continues to be in speech therapy. What I really wanted to say is that I don't really understand what happened, but what I do know is that there is a very big and significant change here.

When there was no hope, you created that change. Healing power came through you to her, and I will always be grateful and indebted to you for appearing in my life at a time when I just wanted to crawl under a rock and die. Thank you.

Dr. Kaye: You are very welcome. I feel like I have just been an instrument for her healing. Could you also comment on your personal experience as I was working on Jane? On one occasion, you were seated in another room and you got quite still.

Mary: Jane was having some problems settling down as I remember. She was running around the room and having some difficulty focusing. I went into a room adjoining your treatment room and I sat in a very comfortable chair. I just began thinking about the two of you. As I sat there with my eyes closed, I began to feel golden particulates that were moving like energy. It is hard to describe, but it was as if there was some magical electrical charge. It was something I had not seen before. As I closed my eyes, the whole space of blackness that I had seen became golden. It was shimmering with glittering particulates. I was out of it. It was as though I was meditating and I was just gone.

What I next remember is that I woke up and the house was quiet. Forty or forty-five minutes had passed. When I peeked into the next room, I saw that Jane was out. She looked like she was out cold. This is not a child who sleeps during the day. She slept after the session, and as a matter of fact, she has slept after most of the sessions with you for three or four hours. It was as if she were having extreme exhaustion. She is just constant energy, so sleep is not her thing.

Dr. Kaye: I experienced her energy. As I recall, before she calmed down she was eating pretzels in the bottom of my closet.

Mary: I see her as being a tornado of life. She is just this ball of energy. She was at your piano; she was moving through the whole house. She had pretzels in her mouth. I struggle with, "Oh my God, my child has all of this wonderful activity and isn't that great, when I expected there to be nothing." Her response [after a treatment] is like getting an animal from the vet who has had minor surgery. She is limp. I take her home and it takes three or four hours for her to come around. She takes a nap and is always peaceful afterwards. She wakes up gently and says, "Hi Mommy." She will have a very quiet evening. Trust me. This is not like her.

Dr. Kaye: Is there a final comment you would like to make?

Mary: There are so many things that I would like to say, and so many things that are important. How do I pare it down to a couple of sentences? It is important for me to say first of all, thank you for your help.

My cognitive mind, my linear mind does not have words for this. There was a time when I couldn't be in this realm. If I didn't have words for it I didn't have any understanding of it. It was outside of my realm of life. What I know now is that when I clear a space in my life for this to be a part of me and understand it, obviously, there are tremendous benefits. I got my little girl back. I got my family back intact.

You know, my husband and I spent months shrieking at each other, and there was so much anger and devastation. What we have back now is a happy, functional family. I don't have words to say what this is about or how to explain it. I know in my heart and I know because of what I see and because of what people say that there has been a tremendous healing and change, and I would just encourage anyone who is skeptical to try it because there was no greater skeptic than me. I'm not into astrology or chakras. In fact, I tend to be in the position of, "prove it to me, then I'll believe it." I allowed this to be and made it OK for myself so that it didn't have to have words. I couldn't understand, but I could describe it. My life has completely changed because of that willingness to surrender to something that is bigger than me.

Dr. Kaye: Beautiful. Thank you so much.

Commentary by Gary Crosby

I was getting really tired of going to doctors, getting more tests, and not getting any better. My friend's son, Michael, was seeing Gloria, and when we visited him we invited Gloria to join us for dinner. I liked her right away. She is warm, funny, and her eyes sparkle when she talks. She is not a quack.

We all sat around the table, and when the conversation turned to healing Michael complained of a headache. Gloria fixed the headache. I was impressed that the pain went away so fast. I talked to Gloria about my aches and pains. I told her that I have a mechanical device that replaced one of my heart valves. I was going on and on about my heart and the noise that this device makes. It was always ticking, and sometimes it sounded so loud to me that I was sure everyone near me could hear it. Then she said it—the one-liner that got me going. She looked at me and in all seriousness said, "I guess you'll never be lonely." We all just laughed and laughed. Great line for a modern-day healer.

That's how I got to know Gloria. I decided that this woman was all right and might be able to help me. I had a list of complaints from here to China. Within six weeks and six sessions most of my complaints had gotten much better or disappeared. For instance, for ages I had a bone spur in my foot. During one of the sessions, Gloria put some oil on my foot. I never even told her about the bone spur. All I did was say that I had pain in my toe when I walked or worked out. She said it's not my toe and proceeded to massage an area below the toe where my bone spur was. Miraculously, the bone spur disappeared and I never had any more pain in the toe.

She worked on my hip and my hands. They have been numb to the point where writing became a problem and they would go to sleep. I also had a problem in my neck that started twenty years ago. Sometimes I would have to take four Advils to get rid of the neck pain, but now it just doesn't hurt anymore.

A few minutes before our last session was supposed to end, I half-jokingly asked her if she could do anything about my voice. My dad (Bing Crosby) had a really deep voice, and I have had to try really hard to get down there. She scanned my body and said, "Maybe," and she wasn't joking. A few more movements of those magical hands and I actually was able to improve my range by one whole tone. This was amazing. She wasn't really impressed but offered anyhow to go on the road with us.

The story doesn't quite end here. As I was getting ready to leave, she asked, "Do you still hear that loud ticking?" I had to think for a minute. How did she know about that? No, the ticking was not nearly as loud. In fact, I couldn't even hear it. I asked her how she knew. She just smiled and said, "Hope you won't be too lonely."

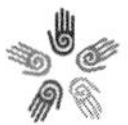

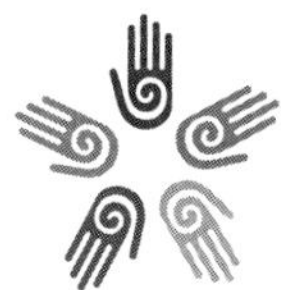

C h a p t e r   3

Various Conditions Treated

Cancer Patients

I have treated many cancer patients and have had physician support in nearly every case.

When someone comes to me with arthritis, migraines, colitis, I'm usually able to assist them within a few short visits, and my success ratio is in the 90th percentile. Cancer is less predictable. Some patients have needed only one treatment, while others have required multiple sessions. One woman that had cancer on the underside of her arm appeared to be responding, but in fact, her doctor told her there was no change. Another woman came to me with some very advanced, ugly open cancers on her breasts. There was nothing I could do to help her. However, it is my inclination to try to help—regardless of the odds.

My former secretary, Amanda, was a cancer patient who had had a hysterectomy. When I first met her she was unable to lift her arm because of a blood clot that had formed where her feeding tube had been placed. I was conducting a group healing, and at the end of the evening Amanda was able to lift her arm up over her head. My work with Amanda had more to do with preventing future episodes than working on the actual cancers. Amanda periodically experienced extreme stress, and I tried to work on her so that future trauma would be negated. Interestingly, she had exploratory abdominal surgery, and when she was opened her surgeon could find no evidence of adhesions or any further cancers. Her surgeon commented that it appeared as if she had never had surgery.

When working with cancer patients it is very interesting to ask about what was going on in their lives six to eighteen months prior to their diagnosis. Stress and/or trauma seem to be the prime factor in the breakdown of the immune system. This failure in the immune system is ultimately the cause of the activation of cancer cells. We all have cancer cells, and, in my opinion, the cells are extremely volatile. They are dynamic rather than in a state of stasis. With this notion in mind, we can begin to see how cancer growth is accelerated. The converse is also true. The proper intervention will allow cancer cells to disperse. The lack of stability in the cancer cells allows them to grow quickly and conversely allows them to transform into healthy cells with the same rapid response.

I frequently have a very unpleasant feeling in my fingers when I touch a cancerous tumor. I currently use a damp compress when working on tumors. The fingers will tingle in a very uncomfortable way, and even washing my hands after a treatment will not necessarily relieve the unpleasant feeling. When my fingers are placed on the tumor with the express intention of reducing it, a vibration is set up and begins almost immediately to change the character of the tumor. The tumor may actually visibly reduce in size, appearing to get smaller in diameter. At other times, the character of the tumor changes; it can get softer, less raised, or lighter in color. In the case of internal tumors, specifically breast tumors, the character can be assessed by palpating the tumorous mass. Remarkable changes can occur in a very short time.

Carolann is a good example of this immediate response. She was identified with tumors in her breasts. She had had a mammogram and was scheduled for surgery. At the end of her forty-five-minute session, we were not able to feel any masses in her breasts. She subsequently had five ultrasounds, and nothing could be seen. I began by working on Carolann's back. The energy in her body was contracted, and by working on her back more energy moved through her body. With better alignment in her back more energy was actually able to go to her breasts. Carolann's secondary complaint, coincidentally, was back pain. In fact, Carolann had a curvature in her spine, and this seems to have disturbed the energy to her body.

After moving through Carolann's body and correcting these imbalances, I was able to actually touch her breasts. By this time, the character of the tumors had changed. When I placed my hands on Carolann's breasts, the tumors were softer and somewhat smaller in size. The energy continues to work on the areas of distress even when I am no longer actively infusing the client. The energy has a far higher intelligence than we mortals, and it will continue to do its cellular work. Carolann has remained cancer-free for several years, and her prognosis is very good providing that she does not experience any undue stress.

Penny's case does not have a happy ending. Penny had a very rare cancer, and after her diagnosis she was given a very short time to live. Surrounded by family and affluence, Penny prevailed for several years. Penny decided on the traditional approach and chose chemotherapy. My services interfaced with her medical treatment. It was a true marriage of disciplines. Penny received her chemotherapy in Cedars-Sinai Hospital in Los Angeles. It was very challenging for me to treat her while she was undergoing treatment. The atmosphere of the treatment center was very pleasant. Fresh fruit was available to both patients and visitors. A huge fish tank with bubbling water was a soothing presence. The nurses were cheerful and accommodating.

The challenge was dealing with the actual chemicals, which pervaded the air. They have no smell and they couldn't be seen, but they were there. The toxicity in the air drained my energy. The toxicity of Penny's body was also draining. Although I was challenged, I chose to treat Penny every week. My decision was based on our commitment to each other and the fact that I was able to calm her while she was receiving her treatment. I weighed the evidence and then took whatever measures I could to protect myself. I was continually drinking water and urinating to rid myself of this toxicity. Many times, I left the cancer center feeling slightly nauseated. I learned that the most effective way to treat Penny was to do long-distance healing on her. I would sit by her bedside and draw my impressions and then use the pendulum to assist with corrections. Penny was very grateful, and I continued to see her.

After about two years of nearly weekly healing treatments, Penny decided she wasn't sure if my treatments were helping her. She decided to suspend treatments with me and unfortunately she went downhill after that. Apparently, my treatments helped Penny to maintain, but we realized this only after the fact.

My first success story in treating cancer was with a Korean engineer who spoke very little English. He had seen my advertisement in the paper, and when I met him in person he had the crumpled advertisement in his wallet. His cancer had metastasized, and I held out little hope for a real reversal. My thoughts were to hold the energy for him and try to help him with his pain. I treated him only twice in his condition, and to my utter amazement his condition totally reversed. His strength returned and he eventually divorced, remarried, and had a child. We lost track of each other, and after five years had passed I received a call from him. His cancer had returned. I traveled ninety miles to see him at his home. His wife and child were beside themselves. They so wanted him to live and recover. I did the best I could, but his Divine plan called for his passing this time around.

My mother passed on April 1, 1999, from complications of breast cancer. The cancer had spread to her brain and caused her stroke. She was taken to an emergency room. I was called by the ER doctor, who suggested that life support be discontinued. I wouldn't agree to that because I've seen so many turnarounds, and I couldn't sign my own mother's death sentence. Mom prevailed for two years and two weeks. Several times during that period, I got similar frantic calls, "Come quickly your mother is dying." Perhaps Mom was dying; however, I would arrive at her bedside and within a day after treating her, she would rally. The energy seemed to reverse this condition. Mom was always very sensitive to my energy, and even at the very end she responded to me.

Surgical Clients

Jane chose to have surgery on her rotator cuff. This is a common procedure, and most surgeons assure patients that this surgery is a benign procedure with a short recovery period. What the surgeons fail to communicate is the fact that the entire body is traumatized with any surgical procedure. Think about the assault the body receives with any surgery. The imbalances that occur from trauma can cause new pain and sensations. Many years can pass and the body can still hold the trauma of the surgery. On many occasions, I have treated clients whose successful surgery left them with pain not specifically associated with the surgical site. For example, after successful lung surgery my client experienced back pain. Another client had successful hand surgery, but she found that her shoulder had become painful when she tried to rotate it.

My preference is to treat a client before surgery and then treat them immediately afterward. When I treat them before a procedure, the trauma seems to be lessened. Treating the patient immediately after the surgery reduces many post-surgical complaints. While still in the recovery room, I treated a patient who had a hysterectomy. I treated her for four consecutive days. The treatment allowed her to walk more freely without clutching her abdomen. Her abdominal distress subsided, and her energy returned more quickly than expected. She experienced no swelling or redness on her incision.

Post-Surgical Experience

Helen was in her early seventies and had just had a hysterectomy. When she was returned to her room her color was poor. I had seated myself in her room about fifteen minutes before her return and tried to positively energize the room and Helen's space through meditation and prayer. Six family members were present when she was returned to her room. I busied myself with Helen and more or less ignored them, although there was tremendous curiosity. Helen was slightly nauseous, and she had abdominal pain. She was put on a morphine drip, and with the morphine and my treatment, she started to relax. I worked on her for two and a half hours, and her color improved; she had no pain and she was resting comfortably.

The next day, Helen was nauseous, had a backache, and complained about a throat irritation that was the result of an intubation tube. This tube is used to keep an open airway. I did two long-distance healings on Helen that day. I called her from my home in Santa Barbara and did healings while she was in the hospital at Cedars-Sinai in Los Angeles. In the morning I worked on her throat irritation, and in the evening I worked on healing her back pain. She was fairly comfortable after the second healing. Her mood changed, and she was in excellent spirits. Her main concern now was her abdominal gas.

Three days later when I arrived at the hospital, Helen announced that she was on no medication. Helen was fairly comfortable; however, she was still bothered by abdominal gas. She had no appetite and walked stooped forward, clutching a pillow to her abdomen.

After a thirty-minute treatment, Helen walked more freely. She actually was walking rather briskly and upright without clutching a pillow to her abdomen. Several medical students and a resident were following Helen's case. Their opinion was that Helen "looked very good."

I saw Helen again the next day. Her abdominal gas was less of a problem, but she was feeling toxic and tense. After her treatment, she was more relaxed and she was looking forward to going home. I was very impressed by the way her incision was healing. She had had twenty-four stitches, and four days after her surgery she had no inflammation. Her incision looked as clean as a paper cut, and she had minimal bloating. This time her internist examined her and announced once again that "it looks good." Helen, in fact, looked almost radiant.

Learning Difficulties

When Linda told me about her daughter, Angel, I immediately got a structural impression of the young girl. The imbalance that I was seeing in my mind's eye was indeed confirmed when I met with Angel. The imbalance in the cranium was causing a split in Angel's perception. It was affecting her vision and her ability to synthesize incoming information. She had difficulty completing homework assignments that involved extensive reading. Angel is an exceedingly bright child, and her difficulty was not related to her intelligence or ability to comprehend; something else was going on with her.

In addition to the irregularity in her cranium, Angel's chin line was not well defined. It was a rather unusual circumstance for a girl of her age. When I pointed this out, Linda said that Angel was born with a cleft palate and Angel had had surgery to correct this condition. It is quite possible that the trauma of the surgery had contributed to the imbalances that I was seeing. In fifteen minutes, Linda and I both noticed a visible change in Angel's appearance. Angel had chosen to close her eyes during the treatment, and at the end of fifteen minutes Angel had opened her eyes. Objects appeared clearer and brighter to her. The change was a result of applying a light pressure to the lower right side of her head. In order to effect a change in the jaw and chin line, I gently stroked the area just below the jaw. I mentally was asking the body to come into balance. The results once again were immediate. Linda and I were able to see a discernable difference in the definition in Angel's chin. As her head settled more comfortably on her neck, the entire structure of her head was altered.

Obviously Angel was very responsive to the treatment. For several minutes we sat quietly as the energy continued to make corrections. I spoke to Linda five days after Angel's treatment. Linda reported that Angel was able to read competently at her grade level. The correction continued to hold, and the definition in her neck continued to maintain. Our next session had its own elements of drama. Angel, being a very active child, never took naps during the day. Twenty minutes into the session, Angel was sound asleep. Linda was astonished. Linda also reported that Angel had continued at her grade level and was preparing herself academically to move into a more challenging school.

Mysterious Ailments

Joanna had suffered for years with chronic dizziness. She was diagnosed with an autoimmune disease and had taken steroids, antibiotics, and antiemetic drugs. She was unable to work and was on disability. From time to time, I am presented with such a complex and emotionally laden situation. There is frequently a sense of desperation and hysteria. The energy surrounding this type of client is particularly challenging. The challenge is to circumvent this energy and connect with the client in a neutral, empathetic manner. Frequently, a client who has had a history of seeing numerous practitioners needs to talk about fears, frustrations, and a sense of hopelessness. When this occurs, I do not immediately place my hands on the client. Listening carefully to the story, but with detachment, I frequently look to the left of the client. It helps me to synthesize the situation and lets my intuition become even more active. The effect of the client can be a distracter when I am trying to make an intuitive assessment. In other words, if the story is told with anxiety, sadness, or elation, it can be very distracting. I try to listen with the third ear and witness the story with the third eye. Joanna was a very brave soul who was trying to weather her storm with equanimity and dignity. As I listened to her story, I saw the inside of her skull. My vision was one of layers of cobwebs. I didn't need to interpret what I was seeing. I was only interested in clearing the area. Working on the neck, I was able to clear the denseness in her skull. Her vision, which we had not discussed, cleared, and the dizziness subsided. When I asked her to focus on an area across from where she was seated, she commented that everything seemed brighter.

I explained to Joanna that I couldn't predict just how the body would react to the treatment. Sometimes the treatment holds indefinitely while at other times the corrections are short-lived. The important thing to remember is that if the treatment was successful in creating a change in symptoms then it would be ultimately successful. The body frequently needs re-education as to what balance is. When an individual has experienced a long-standing imbalance, the body becomes accustomed to a state of imbalance. Corrections will increase the state of balance and the body will then become adjusted to a healthier balanced state.

I explained this to Joanna along with a time-honored notion of recovery. Symptoms seldom resolve permanently and fully with one treatment; therefore, it is helpful to consider this construct. When one is recovering, duration, frequency, and intensity become the barometers of change. For instance, with pain, depression, or systemic complaints one needs to ask, "How frequently am I having symptoms? What is the intensity of the symptom? How long does the symptom last?" This concept was very helpful for Joanna. She was not symptom-free, but her dizziness was not as frequent or intense nor did the episodes last as long as usual. Think about a time in your life in which you were recovering from some challenging episode. Wouldn't it have been miraculous if difficulties were ameliorated spontaneously? It is just not that way. When we begin to look at recovery it is a good idea to look at these parameters.

Joanna's second session was equally delightful. She reported that her dizziness was not nearly as pronounced, although it was still present on occasion. I again treated her neck. Once again, her vision and dizziness cleared. My original vision of the cobwebs had totally cleared and the inside of her skull looked healthy and normal.

Joanna's next visit was a disaster. Her symptoms had returned, only they were not as pronounced. Her color was poor, her eyes looked haunted, and she asked if I could just do what I did during the first session. This request sounded like a reasonable one because we were so successful with the first session. However, placing my hands as I did on our first session was not the answer. What happened between the last session and this session to cause a return of the dizziness? This called for some serious investigation. My instruction to Joanna after our last successful session was to continue her life as she had done in the past without any change. Clients need time to stabilize after a treatment. I often use a visual example of cells stacking up on one another. Healthy cells have a new character, and they interface with each other differently. This new interaction is unstable, and the goal is to create stability with the new cellular structure.

Many times, symptoms will disappear and clients will want to engage in more challenging tasks such as cleaning the closets, taking up an exercise program, or taking care of business. In Joanna's case, I did not mention that changes in diet and medication might affect her progress. This was an omission on my part. Joanna dramatically changed her diet and included more fruits, vegetables, chicken, and dairy products. Unfortunately, Joanna did not realize that inorganic vegetables, fruit, chicken, and dairy were going to be exceedingly toxic to her body. The bovine hormone present in inorganic milk is exceedingly toxic, as are the pesticides on fruits and vegetables. Inorganic chicken frequently poses many problems for the sensitive individual. The chemicals present in commercial chicken are exceedingly toxic. Using the pendulum, I was able to verify my suspicions regarding these inorganic products.

In addition, Joanna discontinued her medication. Joanna had been using scopolamine patches to help reduce her dizziness. When she was symptom-free after her treatment she assumed that she could stop using her medication. Unfortunately, with certain drugs, immediate cessation of the drug can cause a rebound effect. This basically means that even though an individual is symptom-free the immediate cessation of medication can cause the symptoms to recur. I experienced this with a physician who was self-medicating himself for migraines. He was totally symptom-free and stopped his medications. The symptoms reappeared, and he believed that the treatments were ineffective until he considered the rebound effect that may occur with the sudden cessation of medication.

Joanna and I discussed the implications of her situation. She agreed to ingest only organic fruits, vegetables, and milk. She also started using her patch again. I suggested that she increase her water intake, as I suspected that she would be releasing many toxins from her body. I saw Joanna the next day and she was once again symptom-free. She also said that she had been urinating profusely and felt that she had released many toxins. She was feeling lighter and brighter. We talked about the Scopolamine usage and agreed that Scopolamine in tablet form might be more agreeable for her. Her skin had been irritated by the patch. She called her physician and made this request.

I saw Joanna the following week. She came into the office bright and perky. She reported virtually no symptoms. As she described her situation she said, "I might get an occasional twinge, but I don't even pay attention to it." She had lost an additional three pounds. She was looking forward to returning to work, and her fear of her symptoms returning had been totally dispelled. An interesting outcome of this session was to have discovered how an emotional shock to her body had played a part in the development of her symptoms. Shocks of a physical, emotional, and psychic nature can affect skeletal structure. This "mysterious" disease now had a possible origin and we explored additional emotional trauma. She was looking forward to returning to work and felt secure that she would remain symptom-free. We agreed to see each other monthly for maintenance. Joanna was kind enough to document her experience with me. Her letter follows:

Dear Dr. Gloria,

Stop me if you've heard this one before. What do you call a person who for over a year had visited a plethora of doctors, took a myriad of medications, and still spun dizzily like a top?

Answer will be found at bottom of letter.

Tests showed my erythrocyte sedimentation rate at a whopping 85+ (normal is approximately between 12-18), which signified severe inflammation. However, with the reading of all other tests normal, a troupe of baffled doctors had diagnosed me with a mystery autoimmune disease, one which a relief for my dizziness proved quite elusive.

The onset of my illness began very suddenly in October of 1999. Constant, chronic dizziness, and nausea along with severe ear pain and pressure set in with, as far as I was aware, no rhyme nor reason. Months followed with increasing symptoms as many medications were tried and many tests performed. Detrimentally and inconclusively.

In January of 2001, my doctors were in agreement that they would put me on a chemotherapy-related medication along with prednisone. "A mask, not a cure," they said. This was deemed their last resort.

Charles Dickens wrote, "It was the best of times, it was the worst of times…" Obviously, Mr. Dickens, that little optimist, wasn't on prednisone when he penned those words. As I had previously experienced three nightmarish trials of prednisone during much of the year 2000, I was not ready for this kind of treatment. In addition to the prednisone not diminishing my original symptoms, at different times in the past year while on the medication, I had experienced weight gain, difficulty breathing, severe heart palpitations, chronic fatigue, "brain fog," euphoria, and depression. These are just a few of the many side effects prednisone gifted me with, so I was by no means ready to give it another go.

Instead, I asked my rheumatologist to give me a prescription for scopolamine patches used for motion sickness, the only thing that ever gave me relief. Although this relief was welcome, I could only wear the '3 Day' patch for up to three hours maximum, as the adhesive gave me irritating rashes. Taking a patch off and putting it back on later, I found the potency of the medicine greatly diminished. The same with cutting a patch in half…the second half would be very ineffective. In addition, my insurance company only allowed me four patches a month, a small amount that created very few dizzy-free days. It was at this time, Dr. Gloria, that I began sessions with you.

At first meeting, I knew that you were a person I needed to know and that your healing room, scented lightly with citrus, was a sanctuary I needed to be in. To breathe in.

From our first session on, I immediately felt calmed in your presence and soothed by your feather-light touch. Although I've been to see you for the past few weeks, only at our most recent meeting did I realize that you didn't have music playing in your healing room. Even now I can't think of our sessions without hearing a soothing melody.

In the few sessions we've had, I've recognized a gradual change in my health and in my whole being. My dizziness is diminishing and is the only symptom of illness I know to this day. During our healing sessions, it is completely nonexistent. This is the very miracle I had wished for in my going to see you, but you've helped me with so much more! With your assistance, I am no longer on rash-causing patches, as you have since contacted my rheumatologist and worked with him to obtain my medicine in pill form…enough to cover a full month with refills if needed! Also, diagnosed at an early age with migraines, I was taking 3-4 headache pills a day. Since our sessions, I've only been taking that many (if that many) a week! This isn't all…for years as a food addict, I've been struggling with my weight, never able to lose any, but have had great success in gaining! 'Til there was you. A few weeks ago you suggested a diet of organic foods and helped me write a grocery list of the foods that are best for me. On this day I am pleased to say that I no longer think of food as convenient comfort but merely as occasional sustenance, and cravings are now alien to me. All in all, I'm feeling much healthier. I'm standing straighter, I'm losing weight, and I'm enjoying exercise for the first time in a long time!

So, back to the riddle at the beginning of this letter. You have taught me that what's important is not necessarily finding the diagnosis of an ailment but rather searching for the cure. We are well on our way!

With great appreciation,

Joanna

P.S. One last note about our sessions…you speak such words of encouragement during a treatment that I get a glow of pride in feeling that I'm doing something wonderful. How can this be when you are performing the magic? Credit should be given where credit is due. Gloria…Alleluia!

Back Pain

Back pain is frequently associated with imbalances in the back. When these imbalances are corrected, the pain usually subsides. I treated a woman who had back pain for several years, and her doctors couldn't determine what was causing her pain. This patient had had foot surgery and by favoring her left foot, she had created imbalances in her back. Although the surgery was successful, she was left with a sensitivity in her fourth toe. Walking had become a very painful event. She was used to walking twelve to fifteen miles per week, and she depended on the physical exercise to keep her weight and depression under check. Because she was no longer able to take her long walks, she ate when she felt depressed. It became a vicious cycle. She gained weight, and that caused her feet and back to hurt even more.

By correcting the imbalances on the left side of her body, her foot pain subsided. At the end of her first session, she put on her tennis shoes and tested the condition of her feet. She had no pain and walked confidently out of the office.

The basic premise holds true for chronic pain. John is a seventy-four-year-old who had back pain for the last twenty years. He had had six unsuccessful back surgeries, and his pain only intensified. He had begun self-medicating with alcohol and was now abusing the substance. I treated John for about three months. His pain was nominal at the end of this time, and he was able to work in his garden and prune his trees. My approach to his treatment was the same as it is for acute cases. I try to assess the imbalances and find the places in the body that are available to receive energy. When I find these areas it is like putting a key in a keyhole and unlocking the door. The energy will move and spread in the body to areas where it is needed.

Scoliosis is another condition that can be painful. The skewedness in the spine causes many imbalances. Kelly is a seventeen-year-old who had severe pain in her left shoulder as a result of scoliosis. After treatment she was virtually pain-free, and visually her back appeared to have only a slight curve.

Kelly was recently involved in a serious automobile accident. She was in pain as a result of the accident. Within two weeks after the accident, she was once again pain-free. Her ability to recover as rapidly as she did is an important consideration. If she had not been treated prior to her accident, the additional trauma to her body would have remained with her for a longer period of time. Due to the fact that her spine had corrected, the trauma of the accident did not leave an indelible imprint on her.

Problems with the Feet

Bunions and bone spurs are two of the more intriguing conditions that respond well to energy. It usually takes six treatments to completely reduce bunions, but after the first session most individuals experience increased comfort in the joints of the big toe. Women can sometimes wear shoes that they were previously unable to wear after just one session. In all cases when treatment is complete, clients are able to walk without pain and wear a greater variety of shoes.

When the feet become problematic, so many nuances need to be considered. The arches may need attention, the metatarsal may need to be enlivened, and the entire character of the foot may need to be addressed. Frequently after foot surgery, areas that have been traumatized present a situation of deficit. The color, character, and density of the foot may have been affected by the surgery. These subtleties are difficult to describe, but it is similar to the difference between a sunny, crisp day and a foggy, gray day. Feet have a tendency to quickly respond to an energetic treatment.

It is possible that because the feet have many nerve endings, the conduction of the energy is more expedient.

By gently touching the ankles, I have seen the entire character of the foot change. The color may become rosier, and the arches may become more pronounced. Many times, the foot will hold trauma even though the foot has not been directly traumatized. A very good example of this is the "shorter leg syndrome." Clients have frequently been told by other practitioners that one leg is shorter than the other. In most cases, the shorter leg is actually the result of an imbalance in the hips or pelvis. When the skewedness in this area is pronounced it can give the appearance of having one leg shorter than the other. When the higher hip is adjusted by infusing that area with energy, the legs appear to be more similar in character and length. Usually, the higher hip will also be holding an over-energy. This not only creates a deficit in the opposite side, the over-energy also creates an unwanted tightness in that area. It is interesting to have the client stand after the connection is made. It takes a few seconds to get used to the feeling of balance and the way in which both feet are equally supporting the body.

I believe that bone spurs sometimes form in the feet as a result of an imbalance. Parts of the foot are overused when there is an imbalance. This imbalance causes additional pressure in one area of the foot, and bone spurs are more likely to occur in those areas. To relieve, reduce, and eradicate bone spurs, the logical step is to create more balance in the body. When the weight of the body is more evenly distributed, the weight will be carried more evenly in the foot. In the case of the bone spur, after the entire foot has been enriched with energy, I will work directly on the painful bone spur.

By applying a gentle pressure along with an intention to transmit energy, there is usually a softening under my fingertips.

One of the more interesting situations that relate to balance was the case of Jack. His advanced diabetes created diabetic ulcers in his feet. Jack's right foot had a stubborn open sore that would not heal. He had tried antibiotics, topical creams, and various implements in his shoes, but his ulcer prevailed. Jack's body was out of balance, and he placed more weight on his right foot. One of the reasons his ulcer was unable to heal had to do with the fact that every time he took a step, he put more pressure on his right foot than the left one. Every time he took a step he further irritated his condition.

By correcting the imbalance in Jack's hips, he was able to exert more balanced pressure on his feet. The energy was also able to lift his arches and further reduce the pressure on his feet. The results of this work were especially dramatic.

Another interesting aspect of this healing had to do with the fact that Jack's blood sugar was affected by the treatment. Jack frequently monitored his blood sugar, and he invariably discovered that this blood sugar was lowered after his treatment. Whether this was a result of the relaxing effect of the treatment or this somehow affected him systematically, we may never know. However, many of my clients who have diabetes found that they were overall using less insulin to keep their diabetes controlled.

Migraines

Migraines can be a difficult and complex situation to address. By the time I treat a client whose primary complaint is migraine, that individual has usually seen many other practitioners. The complaint is usually a long-standing one. An emotional overlay associated with pain and a compromised lifestyle is frequently present. A number of considerations must be addressed at the onset of treatment.

What physical imbalances exist with this client? I naturally consider imbalances in the cranium, but other imbalances in the body can also contribute to a lingering migraine situation. What components contribute to the condition? Was there a trauma, either emotional or physical? How has the pain experienced by the client interfered with the activities of daily living? What environmental stressors are contributing to this situation? Environmental stressors may include air pollution; mold; fabric softeners; personal products such as shampoo, toothpaste, and/or food sensitivities.

As you can see, this is a complex situation but does not necessarily require extensive treatment. Quite frankly, my psychic abilities cut through much of the unknown. For instance, I usually get clear information about the age of the client when the initial trauma occurred. I zero in on the age and the client is usually able to identify the offending trauma. My psychic abilities are also very useful in identifying the environmental stressors associated with the complaint.

Physical imbalances are the most major culprit in the causation of migraines. There are many reasons for these imbalances; however, just correcting the imbalances frequently gives immediate relief.

A young teenager whose parents had recently separated developed migraine headaches. She had no history of any problems with headaches; however, she had an identified scoliosis. The imbalance caused by the scoliosis became more pronounced as the emotional climate became stormier. The additional stress to her body added to the irregularity in her neck. The curvature in her spine went to her neck, and with the increased emotional involvement, her neck became contracted. By making an adjustment in the neck, it changed the flow of energy to her head and she got immediate relief. In this young woman's case, she was unwilling to address her emotional turmoil, and even though she experienced relief, I would have felt much more comfortable continuing treatment. Later, I learned that her migraines had ceased and she only had occasional headaches.

Emotional factors frequently play a role in the etiology of migraines. It is my belief that shocks to the nervous system contribute to the development of migraines. One client who had a twenty-year history of migraines was able to trace her onset to a traumatic event. Her family suddenly experienced unusual financial setbacks. They were destitute and hopeless. Within a year after her trauma, she developed disabling migraines.

My explanation for this delayed onset has to do with the body holding onto prolonged stress. Her body became accustomed to tension and the imbalances resulting from tension. Her cranium became involved and the pain on the right side of her head persisted. Her recovery included discovering the offending event and reducing the strength of the memory of the event. We also made adjustments in the cranium and created greater balance with her skull.

Environmental factors can be slightly more elusive. It is some-times difficult to isolate offending airborne stressors. Generally, ocean air has less pollutants and irritants. Unfortunately, bright, sunny, seemingly innocuous days can heat up hydrocarbons in the air. This is a very difficult situation for individuals who have sensitivities. The heat of the day potentates the pollutants.

I have found that food sensitivities can also exacerbate symptoms. Food sensitivities can vary from individual to individual but basically additives and preservatives in food are very offensive to migraine sufferers. Vitamins can also cause adverse reactions. If you find that you can't assimilate vitamins, spray vitamins might solve that problem. Scented products which could include body washes, clothing detergent and or fabric softeners are also very toxic to the sensitive individual.

In most instances, migraines respond well to energetic healing. Many individuals who suffer from migraines have pronounced imbalances in the face. Frequently the neck will be tense and skewed to one side. Most cases of migraine headaches will respond in one to five sessions.

Larry, who is a real estate developer, has had relief from his chronic pain, and states:

"After twenty years of pain and suffering from almost daily headaches, and after having exhausted all conventional remedies without success, Dr. Kaye freed my body from headache pain which, on reflection, is a rebirth."

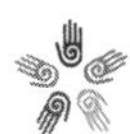

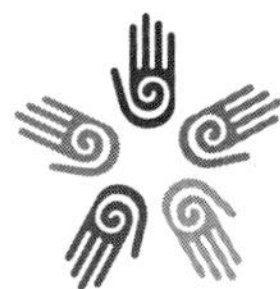

C h a p t e r   4

Holistic Care For Elder Angels

My idea for a holistic-oriented center for elders had been germinating for some time, and in 1988, Casa Glorietta was established. After extensive negotiations, I became the sole proprietor of an 8,500-square-foot building with twenty-five rooms and twelve bathrooms. I was never much into domesticity, so my lessons came quickly.

My first mission was to give this ordinary, drab facility some life and pizzazz. I wanted Casa to be lively, so I decorated the hallways with costumes and posters of movie stars. I quickly made history of the endless, boring corridors. A huge lavender ball gown, long gloves, and a poster of *Gone With the Wind* tacked to the wall created an impression of a time long gone. Another whimsical piece with a Western motif portrayed a cowboy and cowgirl. I visited our local thrift stores and found jeans, jodhpurs, boots, and hats that would set this mood. We nailed some wooden planks to the wall, creating an instant corral.

I was able to acquire a thirty-five-foot mural that depicted scenes of Santa Barbara. This huge piece fit beautifully at Casa and definitely made the corridors less bare. Each five-by-seven-foot panel told a bit of the story of Santa Barbara. Casa was taking shape and having an artistic, creative ambiance.

Casa Glorietta became a family affair, and employees brought their kids, grandchildren, aunts, uncles, cousins, sisters, and brothers to visit with each other and with the elders. As a perk, I offered my services to the families of my employees. Within a short time, the energy there was distinctive, and visitors would invariably comment on how good the center felt. My friends would visit sometimes just to "hang out." It was quite a tribute to experience this feeling of intergenerational community.

The meals at Casa were very special. Having an interest in good nutrition, I was committed to serving meals that I wouldn't hesitate to eat. At the beginning of the project, we bought fresh fruits and vegetables daily. Our breads were commercial but made from organic flours. The only canned goods we stocked were tomato sauce and tomato paste. There were no salt shakers on the tables and very little salt was used in our cooking. Meals were generally low-fat, and our baked goods were monitored for low sugar content. Our storeroom was virtually empty except for staples such as brown rice, potatoes, corn meal, and flour. (We used the storeroom for stashing our art supplies.) To avoid using preservatives, I had everyone involved in food service reading labels. I was like a new mother unwilling to compromise her brood. The cook and I had more than one heated discussion about not using onions and garlic in the cooking. Even though garlic is supposed to have many wonderful curative properties, my experience has always been that sensitive, elderly individuals have difficulties with this bulb.

It was quite interesting to see the changes that took place with newcomers. Within a few days after joining the community, many of them would begin to emit an unpleasant body odor. This lasted for a week or two while the body cleansed and detoxified. The reduction of preservatives, excess fat, and refined flours seemed to stimulate this process. Residents were much healthier and problem cases of constipation were reduced. Along with these changes, some residents became more active and exercised in an outdoor walkway.

Each resident had a primary care physician, and many of the physicians who were involved in caring for this brood were extremely supportive. In many instances, we combined natural interventions along with Western medicine. For instance, during the flu season, we used ginger compresses along with pharmaceuticals for coughs, bronchitis, and upper respiratory conditions. We used massage for constipation and homeopathy for mild diarrhea. With the attending physicians' orders, we used herbal remedies to combat depression and anxiety. The elders perked up and rejoined the human race.

One resident had periodic episodes of painful arthritis. She would wince as she walked along the halls and, at times, wasn't even able to get out of bed without assistance. She nearly always responded to the energy work along with remedies that we used for arthritis. It was just a matter of days for our natural remedies to take effect and produce positive results.

This ideal situation lasted for several years, and then a change in state evaluators forced us to alter our menu. We were no longer able to have daily supplies of produce; it was mandatory that we have a three-day supply of perishables on hand at all times. The art supplies in the storeroom were replaced with hundreds of cans of food. Beef stew, pork and beans, and chow mein were some of the main dishes that the evaluators were pleased to see. Planned desserts of Jell-O and canned fruit filled and contaminated the shelves. My intention to properly nourish my elders was completely undervalued. Even though I recognized the need to be prepared for emergencies, it was very difficult for me to look at rows and rows of canned food.

Because I wanted my elders to be stimulated in every possible way, something was always going on. For years, I had supported a Tibetan child, and when it occurred to me that my elders might enjoy corresponding with Tashi, we all adopted him as our child. We had a framed corkboard where we posted his picture and all of his correspondence. He used to send us letters and his report cards. It was always a treat to receive his correspondence. We made it an event when Tashi's letters arrived. They were always so colorful and touching. The following is an excerpt (unedited) from one of Tashi's letters:

> *Our school is a bordering school. It is 150 km far away from my home. The place where our school settled is named Dhalhousie. This place is one of Hill Station in India. So many tourist visit this place because of its elegant view from the hill. Climatic condition over here is pleasant.*
>
> *Every way flowers blossom, Cold Summer breeze coming from Sea. Made Bough of tree waving like anything as it says come here. Water nipping in the golden light. Any way it seemed very beautiful.*

I am very happy in my school. Lastly I pray to god for your long life and may success what so ever you do. you are very graceful for me same as my parent. I love you and millions of Kiss from me…

That's all.

Yours loving Son Tashi dorjee

Casa became a hub for international correspondence. On one of my trips to Costa Rica, I visited with an American who was organizing a Montessori school in the little jungle community of Puerto Viejo. Sally and her beautiful five-year-old daughter lived in very primitive conditions in this coastal village. Wanting her daughter to be well educated without leaving Costa Rica, Sally created a Montessori school where both her daughter and other village children could attend. It was a huge undertaking, but Sally located a building that was suitable for classrooms and proceeded to develop the Montessori model. The children began corresponding with us and one of the first items we received was a collage of Costa Rican foliage from local trees and shrubs. We created a separate area for displaying the work of these children. Our elders responded by sending drawings that they created in their art classes. This monthly exchange of drawings and letters was stimulating and helped reduce feelings of isolation. Through international contact, residents who participated in these projects felt the expansion of Casa's borders and part of the world community.

Because we attracted many artistic individuals with rich histories, I decided to develop Casa as a showcase for senior community art. Our first exhibit consisted of over sixty underwater scenes created by a local senior artist. These lovely pieces had a certain whimsical quality to them, and the artist was very pleased to have space to exhibit so many pieces. We had over fifty guests, and our elders appreciated the art. All of the elders enjoyed the lively interaction with the guests.

Our second show posed some problems. The state regulators were concerned because no care home owner had ever had ongoing art shows. When they fully examined their regulations, they decided that I was in violation of Title XXII. The following is an excerpt that appeared in a local paper, *The Independent*, on March 28, 1991:

> *...in the opinion of the State Department of Social Services Licensing Program supervisor, "Art Happenings" violates part of the California Code of Regulations which state that each resident 'shall be accorded safe, healthful and comfortable accommodations, furnishings, and equipment.' According to the supervisor, this rule is relevant to the art shows at Casa Glorietta in that the residents' privacy could be invaded by 'members of the public wandering around the halls.' A (second) display of works by senior citizen painters... had to be canceled due to the Social Services ruling.*

Supporters of Casa were outraged, and we received many letters of support. The main theme of the comments had to do with the State's interference with an uplifting, positive presentation. Many individuals wrote directly to the State. After all of these years, people still stop me and remember Casa and the art shows.

Here are excerpts from three support letters:

> *...[State officials are] incorrect in ruling that it violates State of California Code of Regulations which states each*

resident 'shall be accorded safe, healthful, and comfortable accommodations, furnishings and equipment.' You give all of this to your patients and more. The showing of art does not affect or create any problems for your patients from what we saw at your previous showings. The patients enjoyed the paintings and so did the visitors.

…The family and friends of V. B. (a patient) are very disappointed that Casa Glorietta has been asked to remove the wonderful art work. It is not only bright and cheery but gives the clients a feeling of pride. What possible harm can it do to provide a warm atmosphere instead of a cold sterile one?

…My mother and I visited father constantly, and our experiences were that he and all the other patients were pathetically happy to see `outside' visitors walking around, instead of just the uniformed workers. Other patients would always talk to us, sometimes gibberish, but it was obviously a meaningful social contact for them. Sometimes they'd touch us, and follow us around as we walked with my father. Several would habitually sit on the front porch, and perk up when any car drove up, and rise to greet anyone, and then 'help' people in the front door.

…My father was in several other places before he died, and, from this experience, we know he got much better care where there was a high visibility to the patients and lots of visitors. There is a paucity of visitors in these places, and Dr. Kaye is greatly to be commended for coming up with a novel way to get more people into her facility. If a resident wants privacy, the rooms do have doors, but humans are far better served to be included in normal social contact rather than being forcibly isolated from it.

And from the exhibiting artist…

…Thanks so much for the privilege of exhibiting my paintings at Casa Glorietta. You and your entire staff were most gracious to me throughout the time of hanging and showing my work. Again, thanks for the honor of showing my paintings at Casa Glorietta. I appreciate it greatly and certainly commend you for bringing community activities to the residents, most of whom could rarely, if ever, get out into the community to attend them. You're doing a great job.

The families of our residents also appreciated Casa and frequently got involved in the care of their parents. Ruth, who was in her nineties, had a very loving, attentive family. They were also wise and knew that she was extremely manipulative. She was also addicted to Ativan, an anti-anxiety medication. With the support of the family, Ruth's physician, and my knowledge of herbs and homeopathy, we were able to maintain Ruth on natural remedies so that she no longer depended on Ativan. Our relationship over the two years that we knew each other developed into a deep affection. Ruth's family wrote a glowing letter of support.

…Indeed a noticeable improvement has been observed by several family members of Grandma's general physical and emotional condition since her taking up the wonderful residence where she now resides. She also is secure within the well run, well managed, clean, quiet, safe building—the close supporting family members feel comfortable with the decision they made last October, 1988 in placing Grandma where she is now—her 'new home' as she has said. Grandma has no regrets and is looking forward to

greater participation on her part in the living, caring and fun at Casa Glorietta.

The Citizens of Casa

Eugene and his wife Lillian were the loving couple of Casa. Eugene used to push Lillian's wheelchair around the corridors looking very gallant when, in fact, the wheelchair served as a pseudo walker for him. Eugene and Lillian were a very spiritual couple and totally aware of my gifts. Lillian had been a psychic reader in her younger days, and she thought of me as a sister. Eugene was a great scholar, metaphysician, and former violinist with the St. Louis symphony.

On one occasion when Lillian was hospitalized and Eugene was in a wheelchair, we took Eugene to the hospital to visit Lillian. When we were ready to leave, he insisted on giving his lady a proper farewell kiss. It took two of us to hoist him out of the wheelchair to reach his beloved Lillian. He kissed her face and looked into her watery eyes and whispered, "I love you."

When Lillian was too debilitated to return to us, she went to a convalescent hospital. Sadly, she died the day she was admitted. I immediately went to the convalescent home when I learned that she had died. They were understanding and allowed me to visit with Lillian. I sat with her and spoke with her as if there were still life in her. I thought I could see her chest rising and falling. I touched her thigh and felt an energy move through me, and then I said good-byes for all of us.

We had a memorial service for Lillian; staff and residents joined us. Each of us paid tribute to Lillian as we passed among us a bundle of smoldering sage. I played *Once I Loved* on my flute. It was an incredibly sad, moving time. Lillian and Eugene had no ties with any living relatives, so our support was essential. Eugene sat with his dark tie, white shirt, and tear-stained face and said, "What would I do without you? You're all I have now."

Evelyn

Evelyn was another dear soul whose family fully supported our work. She was eighty-seven, about 4' 8" tall, and suffered from dementia. She talked incessantly about her past. Her speech was eloquent as she engaged visitors with her Southern charm and her expressed nonstop stream of consciousness. It always amused me to observe new visitors when they met Evelyn. They would converse with her and, after a few minutes, would walk away shaking their heads in bewilderment.

There was one thing about Evelyn that you could absolutely count on. She loved to sing *Stormy Weather,* and she would burst out in song with just a little prompting. She could be rambling incessantly and, with a little prompting, start singing that song. She would go on and on, looking deeply and expressively into your eyes as she sang the line "…when my man left me…" She captured hearts with the beauty of her voice and her charisma.

Evelyn, Eugene, and I did a radio spot together. We were advertising the wonders of Casa. Arriving together at the radio station, Eugene had tremendous difficulty climbing a flight of stairs and needed to rest for about twenty minutes before he could breathe normally. Evelyn was talking to herself nonstop and wandering around the station while I was trying to reaffirm my faith in the process, knowing in the recesses of my mind that everything would eventually be all right.

When we actually did the taping, Evelyn was right on. I lead her into her perennial *"Stormy Weather."* She was delightful. Eugene waxed eloquently about the glories of Casa, and I commented on the good times we all had at Casa. Of course, it was necessary to do considerable editing for this sixty-second spot. We needed to delete Evelyn's ramblings, and although Eugene got his second wind, some of his comments were labored so we had to delete his heavy breathing from the finished tape. When the commercial was aired, it turned out to be a real attention-getter.

Evelyn's children wrote this beautiful letter expressing their appreciation:

When my mother was a young woman, she was very good at music (singing and playing the piano). During her fifties through seventies, music gradually dropped out of her life. But at Casa Glorietta, the staff and several volunteers who dropped by to sing with the residents, have drawn my mother's musical talents out, gotten her singing again, and brought back one of the great pleasures of her life. She not only sings when encouraged by the staff, but at other times as well. When I take her out for trips, I frequently find her singing and humming, and it always brings a smile to her face.

Helga

I decided to go into work earlier than usual one day so that I could practice playing my flute before the start of business. As soon as I arrived at Casa, I rushed to room No. 8. This is the room that I referred to as "the magic room" where I did consulting, massage, and occasionally hung out when the pace got too maddening.

Helga had one of the loveliest smiles you could imagine. She was industrious and constantly entertained herself. She was usually silent except for her occasional German responses. You could find Helga folding laundry, setting the table, and generally appearing to have a mission in life. She was eighty-seven, agile, and frequently could be seen picking up pieces of lint from the floor. She had a wonderful passion for life and liked eyeglasses, especially those other than her own. It was not unusual to see her with her lovely smile wearing a very, very strange pair of glasses. On one occasion, she mutely sat in my office. Our eye contact was broken when she, unceremoniously, opened a gold lame purse, removed a pair of glasses, and put them on. They, of course, were not her own.

When Helga first came to us, she had a dual diagnosis of depression and senile dementia. She was heavily medicated and would have frequent crying bouts. Taking the initiative to visit with staff, she would spend hours in our offices mutely and wisely observing us. We gave her space to be herself and respected her unhappiness. After a while she was hardly ever depressed and took very little medication.

Helga was making her rounds just as I was about to enter my room. She saw me and gave me her lovely mute smile. I invited her into my sanctuary and together we started our day. I assembled my flute and began to play. A few minutes later Helga's face was beaming as she said, "Schoen." Since Helga became demented, she reverted to her native German, speaking English only on rare occasions. "Schoen" translates to "pretty," so I was quite flattered that Helga was enjoying my playing. As I continued to practice, Helga announced, "Primo!" while exhibiting the look of a connoisseur on her face. Her gentleness and appreciation moved me.

My most traumatic experience with Helga occurred on Christmas Eve. It was dinner time, and we couldn't find her. After looking in all of our twenty-five rooms, we agreed that she was missing. Where could she have gone? Helga outsmarted our security system. I alerted her daughter and son-in-law and, along with staff and several volunteers, tried to systematically comb the deserted streets for Helga.

After hours of looking, we decided to pray for her well-being. Soon our prayers were answered. Helga had walked four miles to a nearby motel, where she happened to meet German-speaking guests. We were contacted by the motel and were happily reunited. Helga sat in our dining room and ate a hearty dinner. She was laughing as though nothing unusual had occurred. Personally, I felt like I had been run over by a steamroller.

Rita

Rita was ninety-nine-and-a-half years old and just slightly confused. She was about 4' 8" and wore her glasses halfway down her nose. She had two bottom teeth that protruded from her mouth, and she prided herself on setting her own hair with soft, pink curlers. She also delighted in doing her own mending and wrote letters daily to known and unknown friends. She tended to be protective of the women with whom she shared her dining table and frequently asked for second desserts for her table companions.

Because of the periodic swelling in her right foot and leg, we made an appointment for her to see her doctor. Her leg had swollen to nearly twice its size, and she complained of pain in her right shoulder. The doctor told us that she was old and that she didn't need medication. What did we expect for an old woman?

I was livid. After I calmed down, I began treating Rita's shoulder. She was seated in the dining room and, within ten minutes, announced that her shoulder was feeling much better. When I asked her to raise her arm, she demonstrated an increased range of motion. She then said, "This feels so good. Everyone will want to be sick." I laughed and told her that I would take my chances. Not only did her shoulder respond to the treatment but her foot and leg also improved. The swollen hardness of her leg softened, and I could see the imprints of my thumbs on her calf.

The next day, I continued with my massage treatment. Her shoulder was markedly improved and, consequently, I concentrated more on the calf and foot. During this session, Rita showed her sensuous side. She smiled and said, "This feels soooooo good!" At the end of the session, I was able to get a laced shoe on her foot, which was initially impossible due to the swelling. She was delighted as she took a few tentative steps with my Nike running shoe on one foot and her Daniel Green slipper on the other. She was a beautiful, curious sight to behold. This inspirational woman then turned to me, smiled, and said, "I think I'm getting old."

Jean

I was visiting a friend up north when Jean died. My friend and I had just returned from a delightful dinner when I received a message saying that there was an emergency at Casa. As I dialed the number, I noticed that my heart was not pounding, and there was no surge of adrenaline, which was unusual considering the fact that I had heard the word "emergency." This time, for some reason, I was very calm.

The administrator broke the news to me. She told me that in the afternoon Jean was taken to the doctor because of a cough. Her doctor checked her cough and said that there was no irregularity in her lungs. Her breathing was more rapid than usual so he scheduled her for some tests. Jean's son, John, brought her back to Casa just before dinner, and she took her usual place at the table. She ate well, then, complaining of being tired, she went straight to bed.

Sue, the evening nurse, was making her 7:30 rounds when she found Jean looking quite pale and her body cool to the touch. Sue immediately called "911" and the administrator. The ambulance arrived quickly and the paramedics were directed to Jean's room. Soon after their arrival, they called the Sheriff so that the coroner could examine Jean. Not long after the coroner's arrival, Jean was "pronounced" and her body removed. Jean's son had also been immediately notified.

My reaction totally startled me. I didn't seem to have any particular feelings about Jean or her death but was pleased that everything had gone well and that emergency protocol was properly followed. I had an uneasy feeling. Where was my compassion? Had I been intimidated by the system to such a degree that I, too, was only interested in procedure? I was sickened by the possibility.

I remember sitting with Jean. She used to like to touch my hair and would say as she gently stroked my hair, "Your hair is so pretty." I would kiss her forehead; she would look at me warmly and say, "Sleep tight; I love you."

After Jean had passed, I was cleaning her room and putting her possessions in order. Going through her sad dresses, her sad shoes, and her sad hairbrush, I found a neatly laundered, flowered handkerchief. It looked like it was thirty years old. I couldn't help but wonder how many tears it had wiped away during Jean's lifetime. That's when I began my mourning.

Samuel

When I took Samuel to the doctor for his monthly checkup, he had gained three pounds and was in glowing health for his ninety-two years. His depression lifted, and I decided to take him to visit St. Francis Hospital so that those who attended him, when he was recovering from a stroke, could see this delightful miracle. Samuel was a tremendous hit. We first met with Margo in Social Services, and she was truly delighted to see Samuel. When she saw him, tears immediately came to her eyes as she said, "Samuel, how are you? You look wonderful." I felt like a proud parent.

When I first met this very thin, sad man, I cried. I was introduced to him and he said, "Don't beat me. Please don't beat me." My heart sank as I wondered what had happened to this frail, elderly, dignified gentleman. I was soon to learn Samuel's story. His entire family, wife and children, were killed in the gas chambers during the Holocaust. I could hardly fathom the sheer horror this man had experienced.

One evening after dinner, Samuel came into my office. At the time I was talking on the phone to my daughter. He looked very mournful, and I asked if I could help him. With a pleading voice, he said, "Please don't send me to the gas chamber." He was clasping his hands in a prayerful way and kept repeating, "Please don't send me to the gas chamber. I lost mein wife and mein children. I am the only one who is left. I am Jewish." He started to cry. I told him that I am Jewish as well. We began reciting a Jewish prayer together. He cried again. When we finished the prayer, I offered him a flower. Taking it in his hand and holding it to his chest, he stopped crying for a moment and said, "You are a very nice lady."

I assured Samuel that he was safe here with us and that there were no gas chambers. He slowly became a little less agitated. I excused myself and returned to the conversation with my daughter. She had overheard the entire conversation between Samuel and me and said, "Mom, you have a tough job."

I'm afraid my daughter was correct in her appraisal, yet, something positive happened inside me when I could truly say to Samuel or any other resident, "This is your house now. You are safe here. We will take care of you, not to worry." Casa Glorietta had become a haven in which people could gather and heal themselves. There was a space there for residents to explore many dimensions of their lives. They could look at the past and, perhaps, accept and forgive. They could look to the future and know that they would have support for a full, rich life. They could know that their lives were not over and that they were respected and loved.

The End of a Chapter

In January of 1992, I began to see the handwriting on the wall. I had balloon payments coming up, the economy was depressed, and I continued to have $30,000 of expenses each month. At the suggestion of a friend, I listed Casa with a business broker. It was sad because I didn't want to let go of my baby.

I eventually received an offer from the listing agent, and after countering his numerous ploys we finally reached an agreement. The agony of this transaction was monumental. In a business and personal sense, I experienced conflict, impotence, and defeat. It was one of my life's major traumas.

On March 25, 1993, the new owner was given the keys. I removed the lavender ball gown, gloves, and the *Gone With The*

Wind poster. Bogart, Marilyn, and Clint got retired. The lanterns and checkered tablecloths were removed. The thirty-five-foot mural of Santa Barbara was returned to the art museum, and the cook—with my permission and blessings—acquired his favorite potato peeler.

The Friday before the takeover, I invited friends and supporters over to say their farewells. Many people had been drawn to Casa and needed to feel completion. We began the evening farewell ceremonies with a classical guitar concert. After refreshments, many people left and a group of about ten stayed on. We formed a cadre as we walked through the halls. I led the procession wearing my dress of mourner's white. I carried a bundle of smoldering sage and used the smoke from the sage to cleanse the corridors. We walked in silence except for the steady slow beat of a drum. I was transfixed. My feet felt as if they were moving without much effort. I was floating as if the pain had caused me to disassociate. A little monkey, Wu-Wu, was part of the procession. He watched over us as we moved through this veil. I have no further recollection of the evening. The pain was too intense.

The next day, I returned to say my private good-byes. There were a few odds and ends that I attended to. Feeling more grounded, I asked the cook to take a few parting pictures. Then I got into my car for the last time as the owner of Casa and, from the car window, I sadly waved my last good-bye.

Interviews with Senior Clients

An Interview with Tony

Tony, a lawyer, had a variety of complaints including overall stiffness, neck and shoulder pain, and problems with frequent urination. Tony returned to his native Texas and called for an occasional telephone healing.

Tony: My main problem was that almost anything that I drank irritated the bladder sphincter and therefore I was urinating quite frequently, though the volume was quite nominal.

Dr. Kaye: Since this interfered with your life, how did you manage your days to accommodate your difficulties?

Tony: For one thing, if I drank tea at lunch, I had to make sure that there was a bathroom nearby. I had to be very careful if I had any alcohol; a bathroom had to be immediately available. Even though I had a feeling of urgency, there was very little volume. Soda water would also give me the same feeling of urgency.

Dr. Kaye: That must have been very annoying. You also had other complaints. Could you talk about your shoulder?

Tony: My shoulder was aching at night. Whenever I turned over, pain would wake me up. I would have to rearrange myself in order to go back to sleep. This was more of a problem on the left side than the right. Since the first sessions, I have not had any pain on the right side. The pain on the left side took slightly longer, but it is now completely gone.

Dr. Kaye: I remember that after your first session, you were surprised that your urinary difficulties were improving. I remember running energy through your kidney and bladder areas on your back. Then I felt the need to adjust your hips. You were also on the homeopathic Nat Mur, which balances water conditions within the body. After one week, what was your situation like?

Tony: Two days after our session, I noticed that after drinking iced tea at lunch, I wasn't having the urgency that I had become accustomed to and I didn't need to limit my fluid intake. This happened almost immediately. I think in the eight weeks since we started, I only had to urgently leave meetings on two occasions. This is a very significant change. It is most embarrassing to be in the middle of a meeting and not be able to wait…then the aggravation of having the volume be so low.

Dr. Kaye: It sounds like your urinary problem resolved. And the shoulders?

Tony: One of the major complaints, along with the aching, was that during the night I would be awakened by the pain. I also had a lack of flexibility. The right shoulder healed real well, and the left shoulder was slower. I don't know what that was about.

Dr. Kaye: In my opinion, the difficulty with your left shoulder had to do with your neck. By relieving the difficulty in your neck, your shoulder was able to heal.

Tony: I do remember that when you were working on my shoulders on the second occasion, there was a very specific letting go in the shoulder. I also remember that when you were working on my urinary tract, a lot of movement occurred in my abdomen.

Dr. Kaye: Could you describe that movement?

Tony: Not in good clinical terms. All I can describe is that the left-hand side of my abdomen felt like my entrails were being rearranged.

Dr. Kaye: You felt a lot of internal movement?

Tony: Yes. I also felt heat, although at first I was not aware of the heat.

Dr. Kaye: Do you remember if that was about the time that the back pain resolved?

Tony: The back pain lessened after the first session, and sometime after the second session it dawned on me that there was a substantial shift in my body and that I was getting in and out of the car without any aches. I was also able to sit comfortably in positions that had previously been uncomfortable.

Dr. Kaye: The hips. Please tell me about the kind of pain you were having in your hips.

Tony: Basically, there was limited movement in the hip area. I was unable to sit on the floor, and there was restriction in my movement. I had been carrying around an image of my father and his arthritis and how encrusted he had become. Somehow this has been released. My awareness of my body is less, and it is less now because it works. I don't have to pay attention to my movements. Now there is a fluidity to my movements.

Dr. Kaye: I would be interested in your comments on the process of healing.

Tony: The process is a very, very non-threatening one; it appears to be non-invasive. I am also conscious of psychological shifts that occurred, and it is a very painless, pleasant process.

Dr. Kaye: Were you surprised by the results?

Tony: Actually, I was. I was willing to go with it. I had seen a healer twelve or thirteen years ago in Houston, but the results were not very dramatic. I had seen another healer, but your style is less threatening. I pick up vibrations from people, and I have always felt comfortable with your energy.

An Interview with Erna

Erna was on a trip visiting her daughter and agreed to see me. Erna lives in Canada, and our meetings were limited.

Erna: Well I had really bad pain in my groin and hip area all on the right side; the whole right side was cockeyed. And my neck and across my shoulders also was stiff when I went to shoulder-check as I was driving the car. I couldn't turn my neck anymore to that extent.

Dr. Kaye: How intense was the pain in your hip?

Erna: It was really bad.

Dr. Kaye: How did it incapacitate you?

Erna: If I were to get up, I would have to walk at least four steps before I'd straighten up. And the pain was there all the time.

Dr. Kaye: Did you have pain anywhere else?

Erna: Well, in my arms between the elbows and the shoulders it felt, I presume, something like arthritis, but I don't really know what it was. And my knees were, I thought, arthritic, but that was cured the first session.

Dr. Kaye: Tell me about your knees and what it felt like to be pain-free.

Erna: I just ran up- and downstairs several times. I couldn't believe it. I just felt so much younger.

Dr. Kaye: Do you recall what we did during the first session?

Erna: Yes, as you were working on me, I could feel a fluid movement between my hip and my knee on my right side. Just like something boiling almost.

Dr. Kaye: Did you continue to improve over time?

Erna: Yes, it got better. Every day it seemed to get better. I think after the third day—my knees must have been better before that because everything improved, and I didn't notice it until it was gone for a day or two.

Dr. Kaye: When I saw you walk up and down the steps I was astonished because you were almost at a run.

Erna: Yes, I did. Oh yea. I just go up and down those stairs like a young girl.

Dr. Kaye: We also worked on your chest. What's gone on there?

Erna: The day afterwards, I wasn't as out of breath walking upstairs or up a hill. Before that I was, and I thought it was just normal, and then after you gave me a treatment, I could breathe so much better.

Dr. Kaye: So were you attributing a lot of your symptoms to your aging process?

Erna: Oh, yes. I thought that's what it all was. Yes.

Dr. Kaye: Would you tell me more about that?

Erna: As you get older, you expect arthritis and that's what I was blaming everything on. But obviously, whether it was or not, you changed that.

I'd like to say how I got into this, if you don't mind.

Dr. Kaye: Yes, please.

Erna: My daughter had told me about this before and that she was having you work on her, and it was helping her. That was just part of what she would tell me. Then, when I came to Santa Barbara, I had no intentions whatsoever of having any treatments of anything. She asked me if I would like to have a treatment with Dr. Kaye, and just like that, from somewhere without thinking, it just was right that I should do this. God is looking after me and works through Dr. Kaye I am sure.

Dr. Kaye: We've done three sessions now. Do you have any physical complaints?

Erna: No, no I'm…it's unbelievable, just unbelievable how good I feel. I went on holiday, and when I think of what I was like before I came here and got these treatments, I would have not been able to walk and be as agile as I was when we went to Branson. There's just no way I could have done it. I really thank you.

Dr. Kaye: You're welcome. How about your sleep pattern?

Erna: Just great. When I go home, I am going to be telling my friends about this because to me it's a miracle, and if anybody is hesitant at all about trying it, take my word for it, it's worth it. It's just unbelievable.

Erna: I'm sixty-eight years old and my groin area has been deteriorating for at least fifteen years. I originally went to a doctor. He found nothing wrong. I went to a physiotherapist. They treated me and it didn't help. So, I just attributed it to age.

Dr. Kaye: And you were willing to live with it?

Erna: Oh, yes. I was willing to live with it because that's just the way things are…until I came here and met you.

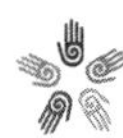

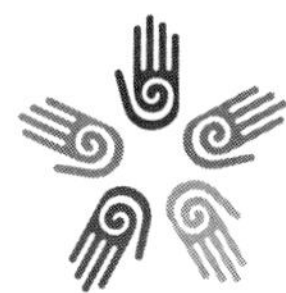

C h a p t e r   5

Animal Kingdom

Wu-Wu

I have found that animal lovers who seek me out are very special, kind, devoted individuals. Diane and her tiny monkey, Wu-Wu, are a good case in point. Diane first called my secretary after our local paper did an extensive article on my work. She was the proud mom of a six-ounce, seven-year-old marmoset monkey. Wu-Wu lived in a handmade pouch that Diane hung around her neck, and in going about her business it was not immediately evident that there was a monkey hanging from her neck. Wu-Wu, ensconced in his pouch, looked like a large pendant.

I was tickled by the entire situation and gladly agreed to see Wu-Wu. When Diane arrived, I was totally enchanted by this little creature. Wu-Wu looked up at me with sweet, darting eyes. Her entire face was about the size of a walnut. Diane explained that Wu-Wu's ability to walk had been affected by what she thought was a calcification in the spine and right shoulder. As a result,

Wu-Wu hopped around, not putting too much weight on her right paw. The right paw toed in somewhat, and the right shoulder was frozen. Wu-Wu also had a serious constipation problem because of her reduced mobility. I had my work cut out for me.

I asked Diane to take Wu-Wu out of the pouch and hold her. Diane began to stroke her, and she calmly responded to the new environment. We both spoke soothingly to Wu-Wu, and I began to stroke her. She immediately looked around with alert, inquiring eyes. We assured her that she was all right, and eventually we transferred Wu-Wu to my lap. It was such a delightful experience. I could feel her relaxing as I continued to infuse her with energy. Her body became very soft as she wrapped her tail around her body to nest. When it appeared that she had received all that she needed, I asked Diane if she would take her from me and place her on the floor so that we could check her progress.

Very slowly, Diane soothingly spoke to Wu-Wu and placed her on the floor. Needing a minute to get her "sea legs," she blinked and tentatively took a step. Within a few minutes, she was freely hopping around. It was a rather remarkable recovery. She placed her full weight on that right paw and hopped around in a balanced manner. She also had several bowel movements on the office carpet as she was hopping around. I had mixed feelings about that, but I was very pleased that her constipation woes seemed to be history.

Diane, Wu-Wu, and I shared many wonderful moments. I met the rest of Diane's family. As they got to know me, they also requested that I see them professionally. Diane's sister, Susan, raised miniature horses, and after seeing the results with Wu-Wu, she invited me to come to her lovely ranch that was home to nearly twenty miniature horses.

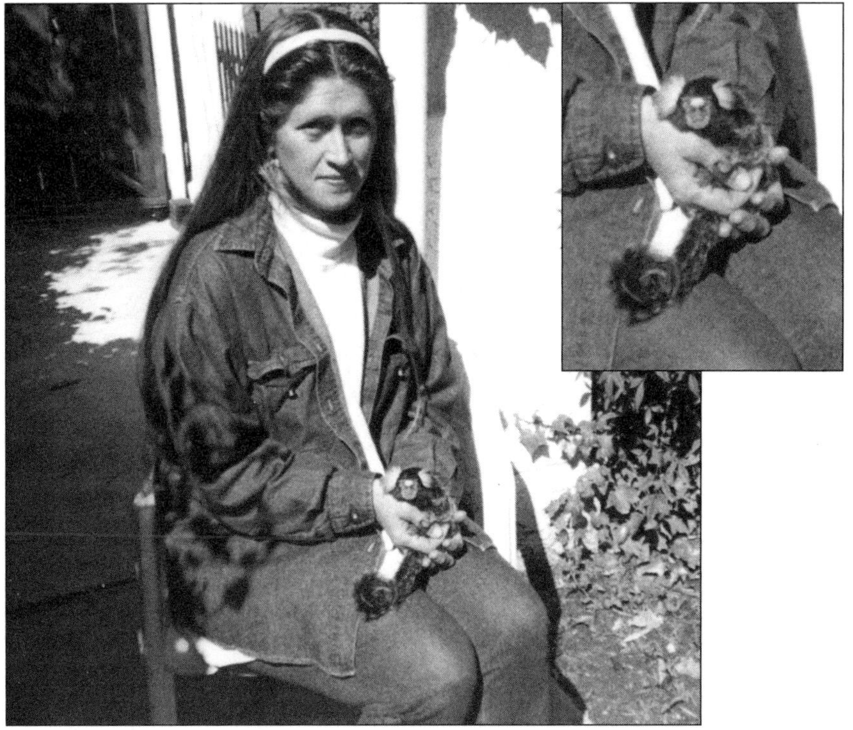

Diane with Wu-Wu

When I arrived at the ranch, I was greeted by a beautiful horse the size of a German shepherd. Susan showed me around this state-of-the-art ranch and introduced me to Inga, one of her Icelandic horses that had foundered. This is quite a serious condition that affects circulation in the hooves, making walking quite difficult and painful. Many times horses are "put down" because of this condition, as medical treatment is frequently unsuccessful.

Inga could hardly support her own weight. She was in her stall on a rubberized surface rather than the concrete surface that would have been unbearable for her. I started to softly talk to her and gently rub her back. She began to relax. Her head dropped, and her body softened as the telltale signs of pain began to subside.

At the end of the session, she was supporting herself more easily. The veterinarian, standing nearby, also agreed that Inga looked at ease. She checked the temperatures of Inga's hooves, and they were more normal. The veterinarian was encouraged by the results of the session. Inga was led back to her personal stall, where she moved with much less fragility and tentativeness.

During my second session with Inga, she was standing well and feeling better, but unfortunately she had developed an abscess in her left rear hoof. Because of the pain she experienced in her front hooves, she put more pressure on her back hooves, causing a large abscess to develop. Susan was attempting to clean it out, but it was so painful that Inga couldn't bear it.

I suggested that I attempt a long-distance healing on Inga, and Susan figured that we had nothing to lose by going that route. I stood about thirty feet from Inga and began to work on the energy fields. Within ten minutes, Inga's whole demeanor changed. She was standing more upright and looked brighter. I suggested to Susan that she try to clean the abscess now that Inga was feeling better. Inga offered no resistance! We were successful in reducing the inflammation. I saw Inga on several other occasions. She recovered well enough to enjoy the rest of her years, even though she was not able to breed or be shown.

Remote Healing: The Mare

Susan was pleased with my work and volunteered to sponsor a workshop on animal healing. It was at this workshop that I met Heather and her daughter, Shauna. Heather was a sensitive, intuitive horsewoman. Both Heather and Shauna were responsive to the energy work, and because of the positive results of the interaction with them and their horses, I regularly visited their ranch.

Their home was nestled in the hills of California's Santa Ynez Valley. As I drove along the lovely winding highway, I marveled at the stunning views. The road to the ranch was called "The Alps" by the locals. Heather also owned property in Kentucky and her racehorses were well known in the industry. I tried not to be intimidated by the lineage of her wonderful beasts, but I have to admit that they impressed me.

I worked on several of Heather's horses during the course of a visit. Although I am comfortable with most animals, I make it a point to have assistance from someone with whom the animal is familiar. Humans sometimes have a hard time describing their reactions to my sessions, so it seems reasonable to have a familiar being close at hand when I work on an animal.

Heather had a few up-and-coming horses with injuries and imbalances. One particular horse raced exceptionally well after her treatment. She came in second in a photo finish. Her stride was beautiful as she moved freely and confidently. In preparation for her second race and to improve performance, Heather asked me to do another healing on her horse. I asked the dates that I would be needed and found out that they conflicted with previously made travel plans to visit my grown children who live in New Jersey.

I told Heather that it would be possible to do a long-distance healing from 3,000 miles away. Heather was willing to try it, so before I left for the East Coast, we arranged for an exact time to connect. Heather drove to Bay Meadows Race Track in Northern California. I was on my way to Newark's airport. As the day of the healing drew near, I prepared my rather conservative, inquisitive daughter by telling her that I would be doing a telephone healing on a horse. She told me that I had been living in California too long, and I countered by telling her that I had learned this skill in Russia.

I gathered the things I would be using during the healing: paper, pen, my pendulum, etc. The telephone rang. It was Heather calling on a portable phone. There was so much static on the line that it took a minute or two to get a good connection. When the line did clear, Heather asked if I was ready for the healing. She was in the stable and, although it was dark, was able to see the significant imbalances in the mare. She was very disturbed by what she saw. She began describing the imbalances starting with the face of the mare. She observed one eye being higher than the other and an imbalance at the nostrils. The girth of the horse was off, and there seemed to be a problem with the left hind leg. I told her we would address one thing at a time and suggested that we start with the face and head.

I made some drawings that I received intuitively, and using my pendulum I began to make corrections. I could clearly hear Heather's sigh of relief as the energy started to correct the imbalances. Slowly, we worked on each of the imbalances that Heather had described. We went through the entire body until Heather was satisfied that the mare was in balance. She thanked me over and over. I made it a point to remind her that this healing had to do with assisting her horse into a space in which she could, in every way, function optimally and that it did not have to do with winning races or money. Heather was in total agreement with this philosophy. Having shared a moment of mutual understanding and thankfulness, we set up a time to speak the following evening.

My daughter had been watching me and listening to the conversation. She commented again, "Mom, come live with us. You have been in California too long." I hugged her and answered that, at the moment, I was riding the crest of a very challenging wave. She looked at me, and in spite of her reservations, I could see that she was proud.

The next day when Heather called I was prepared to do an additional healing. However, Heather was not prepared for me to do a healing. She was laughing too much. I had healed the wrong horse. When Heather arrived at the stables it was very dark. She had not been too familiar with these particular stables and couldn't find anyone to help her locate her horse. She looked into the different stalls and found what she thought was her mare. However, the mare she saw was not hers. The healing I performed was on another mare.

When we both stopped laughing, Heather told me that the horse I worked on appeared to be quite healthy and balanced. I found out later that her mare raced well but not quite well enough to be one of the finalists.

Mary Anne and Her Birds

Not all of the animals I have worked on are four-legged. I met a lady named Mary Anne at a very stressful time in her life. She had raised exotic birds and was a dutiful breeder, hand-feeding her babies throughout the night. She looked like a sleep-deprived new mother, slightly on edge, eyes reduced to slits, and she moved as if she were in a trance.

Mary Anne took me on a tour of her bird community. She had approximately 100 birds, which were in her kitchen, living, and dining rooms. She also had a number of caged birds housed in her garden. Sam was the only outside bird not in a cage. He was a big, beautiful macaw. When I was introduced to him, he immediately nipped at me, a reaction that surprised me. In my experience, birds can only handle a few minutes of energy work. When they have had enough, they let me know through feather and body movements. There was no warning with Sam.

One of the more challenging tasks for me was trying to get the little ones to thrive. Mary Anne fed them around the clock, but some of them continued to have difficulty gaining weight. I studied the chicks in their incubators and wondered how much of this energy would be suitable for beings of one to two ounces in weight? I pondered the subject as I watched Mary Anne tend to the birds. They seemed to like to be held. Mary Anne wanted me to work with a particular chick that was not thriving and had a problem with the digestive tract. I settled myself comfortably in a chair, making a nest with my hands. Mary Anne placed the innocent and wiry chick in my hands. I held the chick for approximately thirty seconds, after which it seemed more alert.

Our next step was to look at the formula that had been prepared for the chicks. I had a suspicion that the formula was too rich for some of them. Through a dowsing technique I was able to verify my suspicions. I made suggestions for the ratio of formula to water. When the formula was presented in a diluted fashion, the chicks began to thrive.

When I returned the following week, they were all gaining weight and looking healthy. Mary Anne was still feeding them through the night, and consequently she was still looking a little piqued. I suggested that she would probably benefit from a short session herself. I felt so much compassion for this woman, whose dedication to her birds was so admirable.

Stephanie the Pigeon

I have also worked with less exotic birds like Stephanie, a poor starving pigeon with one leg. I was introduced to Stephanie and her owner at a dinner party given by my friend Robert. It was a friendly, small party. We were feeling quite festive. As the conversation turned to my healing gifts, Robert's neighbor, Madeline, requested that I try to help Stephanie the pigeon.

Stephanie's feathers were unhealthy looking and sticking up all over. Her little head was tucked into her body, and she was shivering. I needed a quiet place to be with this humbled creature. I asked Robert if I could do the healing in his bedroom. His response was so hysterical that I could only imagine that he had had a traumatic experience with a pigeon when he was a child growing up in New York City. His face reddened, and he vehemently said, "Absolutely, positively no!" I explained to Robert that this was going to be a difficult healing and that I needed a quiet place. He said that he didn't care how difficult it was and that there was no way that I could use his bedroom. I thought for a moment and then asked if I could use his bathroom. Robert softened and looked compassionate. However, the compassion was for me and my desire to work on Stephanie, not for the poor bird. Robert reluctantly agreed to let me use his bathroom for Stephanie's healing.

Stephanie, Madeline, and I entered the bathroom as if we were entering a sanctuary. Madeline seated herself on the toilet seat holding the bird in her hands on her lap. I sat on the bathtub directly across from them. It was a quiet moment, and the only sounds that could be heard were the muffled voices from the party.

I could tell that the bird was going to easily accept the energy, so I instructed Madeline to hold onto Stephanie very securely. I really didn't want to have a pigeon flying around wildly in a small bathroom.

Madeline followed my directions, and within five minutes it appeared as if Stephanie gained about two pounds. Her feathers puffed up, her eyes became alert, and she was now ready to play. Madeline thanked me profusely and wrote the following thank you note:

I have a pigeon who was listless, her eyes were dull and sickly-looking. While Dr. Kaye was healing her, I noticed a gradual but very definite change. She became very alert and her eyes cleared. She would have liked to fly around if I weren't holding her. I saw a very dramatic change in her and after the session she had a voracious appetite. It was a relief to see her looking so much better and eating so well.

Franklin the Reluctant Feline

I had a most intriguing request from a devoted cat lover. Sam and his wife, Tracey, made a point of rescuing damaged cats. Sam had heard of my work and stopped by my office to meet me. He explained that his dear cat, Franklin, was suffering from a bowel disorder and there was little hope for recovery.

I am highly allergic to cats but something about this request caught my attention. I followed my intuition and set up an appointment to work with Franklin. To my chagrin, when I arrived at Sam and Tracey's house, I found myself face to face with eleven other cats.

Sam and Tracey were well known by the Humane Society, which contacted them whenever they were faced with the challenge of a special cat. Their line-up of cats included a three-legged cat, a one-eyed cat, a cat with neurological problems that made it seem intoxicated whenever it tried to walk, an arthritic cat named Pretty Boy, and a variety of other strays.

Sam and Tracey sat on their couch like expectant parents hanging onto every word and suggestion I made. I sat on a dander-free, wooden chair next to the air purifier. They pointed to Franklin, and he immediately retreated behind the television set. They tried to coax him out but to no avail. Franklin was entrenched. My only option was to do a long-distance healing. I always hesitate to use my pendulum on a first visit. Frequently, it's asking a lot to accept the idea of hands-on-healing, and using a pendulum with first-time clients is really an act of faith.

I explained my reluctance to Sam and Tracey, but because Franklin was hiding behind the television, I really didn't have too much of a choice. Surprisingly, they didn't have a problem with my using a pendulum.

When I made my drawing, I could see he had many imbalances and that his poor digestive track was taxed. Usually, I only need to create three impressions and dowse for three drawings. In Franklin's case, there was so much distress that I created at least ten impressions. The information just kept pouring in, and I dowsed accordingly. Finally, it felt as though the healing was complete.

The three of us chatted for a while and, to our surprise, Franklin slowly emerged from his hiding place. It was hard to believe the transformation. Franklin's appearance was totally altered. His legs were supporting him more strongly and, as a result, his torso looked healthier and shortened. He appeared less fragile, and even the texture of his fur improved. He cautiously moved around the living room and found his way to the kitchen. Franklin, who previously had no appetite, was eating voraciously! We were stunned.

When our eyeballs returned to their sockets, Sam asked me to dowse for some pharmaceuticals that he wanted to know about. We did some manipulations and added some homeopathic remedies. I checked on Franklin the following week and found him thriving. This was a cat that was supposed to be on his last leg or on his ninth life, but he was eating well and looking more vibrant. I saw Franklin one other time. This time he stayed on the couch with Sam, and I could quickly infuse him with energy.

Sam was so pleased with the results of Franklin's treatment that he scheduled several sessions for himself. It is not at all uncommon for pet owners to give themselves the gift of a personal healing.

An Interview with a Horsewoman

Paula is an exceptional horsewoman and animal lover. She was born in my hometown of Philadelphia and came from a rather conservative, intellectual background. She is dedicated to her animals and specializes in animal communication.

Paula: I remember talking to you on the phone, and I definitely had a "show me" attitude. We agreed that you would work on one of my favorite horses, Escrow, who had a tracking problem of eight or ten weeks' duration. The tracking problem resulted from Escrow not placing her feet correctly when she walked. I know my mare really well, so I was kind of figuring that I would watch, but I didn't think that anything would happen. As I sat there and watched you work, she visibly relaxed.

Dr. Kaye: What did you see?

Paula: I saw a softness, a dropping of her head; her ears relaxed. Her whole face just seemed happy, gentle, and serene. The muscles in her face, around her mouth, her eyes, her nose just seemed more relaxed. Interestingly enough, I started to experience the same thing, and I didn't want to. I thought it was really strange.

Dr. Kaye: As I recall, you were seated in the barn, watching the healing.

Paula: Yes, at first I was standing in the barn holding her head with the lead rope, and then I sat down because I was getting really relaxed. The mare, at this time, was obviously not going anywhere either. I was not going anywhere. My mare was in heaven, and I started to feel the same way.

Dr. Kaye: At the end of that session, what improvement did you see in terms of the tracking?

Paula: She seemed freer in her movements. She still wasn't tracking perfectly, but she seemed much freer in her movements.

Dr. Kaye: I subsequently saw Escrow for a few sessions, and there was a change in her attitude. Would you describe that?

Paula: Her expression was freer. She was more balanced. Something loosened that was cropped or crimped. She seemed happier and whether her pain was physical or emotional, she no longer seemed to be experiencing discomfort of any kind.

Dr. Kaye: That episode was delightful for me. After that, I worked on Fire.

Paula: Fire got a session because he deserved it. After you worked on him, he relaxed, stretched, pooped, and yawned and stood very tall. Fire puts up with my moods, and this can affect his body.

Dr. Kaye: I remember he looked very bright to me.

Paula: Fire really appreciated what you did. He is my main squeeze; your session was a kind of rejuvenation for him.

Dr. Kaye: I next remember working on Deli.

Paula: Yes, Deli is a gorgeous, 1,100-pound gelding quarter horse cross. He got spooked while he was tied to a trailer, and he jumped. When he came down, he hit his leg on a wheel cover of the trailer. He created havoc, shocked himself, and skinned his knee. He had an attitude and was doing a tough act thing. But anyway, after you worked on him, he just breathed deeply and stretched. His eyes were real soft, and sometimes Deli can get a real hard look in his eye. He is kind of funny.

Dr. Kaye: Paula, do you think that your bad leg and your own jumpiness affected your horse?

Paula: God, yes. I won't ride any of my horses when I know I'm hurting. They pick right up on my pain and discomfort.

Dr. Kaye: After I work on you, what is it like to ride?

Paula: Oh, it is wonderful. I feel so tall and present. I feel at one with my horse, and I ride more freely.

Dr. Kaye: Paula, tell me about your dog's reaction to this work.

Paula: She absolutely loves you. She likes people, but she really loves you. She falls asleep when we're at your house. When I've been over for dinner, she's snored through the entire evening. My dog does not snore. She just does not get that relaxed in someone else's home. I think being around you does for me what it does for her; we both become more relaxed. We both get that same vibe. When I am near you, she gets the vibe by osmosis, and then she is just as happy as a pig in a poke. Her whole expression changes. This is a border collie who is supercharged with energy, and then when she gets around you, she is super-relaxed, and she stretches and her eyes get very soft. It is great to see what she will do with her body.

Dr. Kaye: Can you compare this to any other treatment you have had?

Paula: No. The traditional stuff just doesn't do what this does. I don't know how to describe it. I don't care that I can't describe it. I get lots of pressure to do this the medical way with doctors and vets. I do get frustrated. I am not into drugs for my animals. When you work on us, you can feel the balance. You have to experience this to believe it, and I was very skeptical.

I remember the day Petey got hurt. The big gelding threw his shoe on trail, and the shoe slid back on his foot by about a quarter of an inch and was hitting the real tender part of his foot. He went lame, and he just wouldn't move. His leg was inflamed and swollen when you came to the barn, and within ten or fifteen minutes—with no ice—he was no longer swollen. Very peacefully and quietly, you just worked on him.

Dr. Kaye: I needed to stay very still. He was in a lot of pain and temperamental.

Paula: Oh, he was very frightened. He was not quite ready to go into shock, but, man, he was a scared potato. It was lucky for Petey that you got to him so quickly.

Dr. Kaye: Let me ask you something. If Petey were treated traditionally, what would he have looked like?

Paula: He would have been out for anywhere from two to four weeks. As it was, we let him go easy for a few days, and then it was history. I think that an important aspect of your treatment was the calm that Petey experienced. So much of what is wrong with us physically is controlled by our minds, whether we be animals or humans. My animals trust you. I trust you. You have earned that. I don't want to go to anybody else. I want to go to you, and the animals feel that way, too. Traditional medicine does a lot of drugs and whatnot, and it is not usually necessary. You showed me some things that amazed me. The time I assisted you, when Escrow had a bellyache, was a new experience for me. I think that we all have healing capabilities, but we are so skeptical, and we don't believe our own abilities. I heard her belly respond, and I watched her physically change. She was balanced. She, excuse me, did a really great fart and then a big yawn, and it was then obvious that this horse was not in pain anymore. I would recommend that any skeptic give this a try. This is about balance. You get to stay well by being in balance.

Who-Do

Paula has a hyperactive border collie named Who-Do; she still marvels at the way Who-Do calms down when she is near me. This little dog just doesn't quit, and yet when she comes to visit, she takes on the persona of a big St. Bernard. She just doesn't go anywhere. Paula observed, "When I've been over for dinner, she's snored through the entire evening. My dog does not snore. She just does not get that relaxed in someone else's home. I think being around you does for me what it does for her; we both become more relaxed."

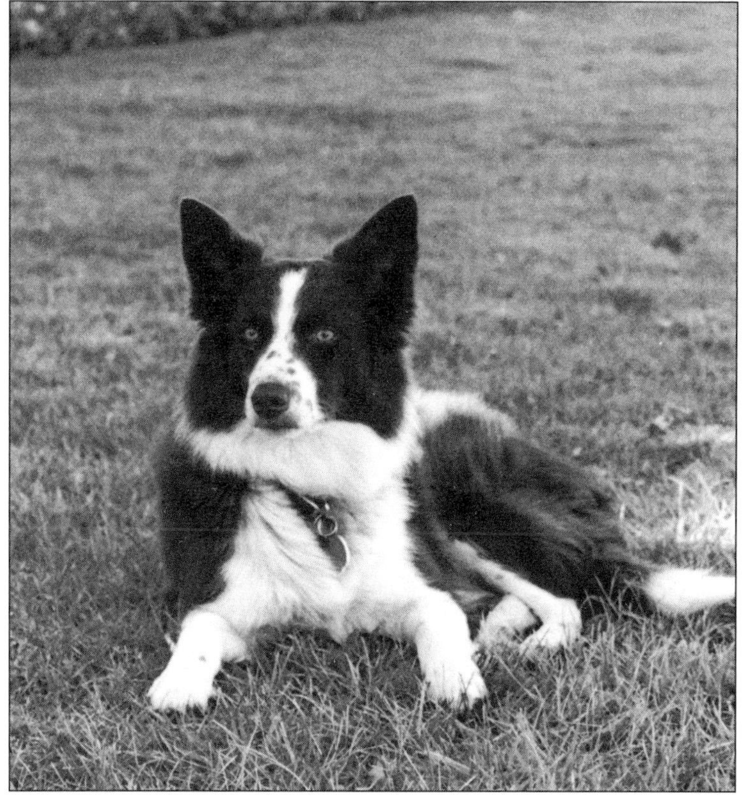

Who-Do

§

The stories are endless and touching, and I find myself in awe of the communion that occurs between human and animals. The animals become our teachers, our friends, and our spiritual kin.

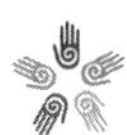

Chapter 6

Scoring High Points With Athletes

"**R**ing."

It was the coach. "Be on the bus at eight o'clock sharp." I grabbed my workout clothes and dashed out into a grey November morning in Oklahoma City. As I scrambled onto the bus, the driver took a hard look at my 5' 4" frame. The rest of the bus was occupied by sixteen half-asleep professional basketball players whose average height was around seven feet. These were the Oklahoma City Cavalry players.

"You're on the wrong bus, lady."

"No. I'm with the team."

This caused some half-asleep heads to turn. I tried to be inconspicuous as I slithered onto a seat, but I was not very successful at blending into the environment. A player named Don swiveled around, cocked his head, and in a menacing voice said, "Coach didn't tell me nothing about a lady on our team."

Was this the time to break the news that these guys were looking at their team healer and yoga instructor? I announced that

I would be instructing the team in stretching exercises that would help prevent injuries. I'm not sure that my diplomatic explanation made much of a difference. I was not looking at a bunch of happy campers.

When we arrived at the gym, the coach was waiting for us. It was the first time I had met him, and he immediately introduced me as the team yoga instructor. There were groans, but the coach countered, "If it is good enough for Kareem, it is good enough for you guys." Kareem Abdul-Jabbar, a highly respected former NBA player, had a long history of injury-free playing. He attributed his flexibility and significant reduction of injuries to his yoga practice.

Well, the news was out. The team was going to learn yoga, and I was the hotshot doctor from Santa Barbara who was going to teach it.

We began our stretches, and to my amazement the team really got into the spirit of stretching and relaxing. Chris, in an interview with the *Sunday Oklahoman*, said, "I've been playing basketball since I was eleven years old. I've played professional for four years, two in France and one in Finland. I'd never done yoga before. At first, I thought it was bogus. I had the idea of wild witchcraft and smoke coming from candles…it is totally different from that. It's mind over matter, and you are in tune with your body. It works!"

After the ice was broken, I announced to the team that I was available to help with their aches and pains. Although my announcement was met with dead silence, after the morning session, several of the players stopped to talk with me and asked about my work as a healer. They wanted to know what I did and how it worked.

I explained that, in many cases, I am effective in reducing pain and inflammation, and in speeding up the overall healing of injuries. I also explained that the touch of a healer rearranges the cellular structure and/or may disperse unhealthy cells.

The guys seemed satisfied with my lecture, and Meyer volunteered to be my first patient. He was soft-spoken; his light green eyes were very innocent and open. Meyer's complaint centered around his neck and shoulders, as he appeared to be carrying the weight of the world on his shoulders. His head and neck were forward, and his shoulders were somewhat slumped. Meyer was a new father and worried about being able to support his family as a professional athlete. We talked for a short while, and then I began to work on him.

I stood behind Meyer while he was seated in a chair. He immediately began to relax. He described a vibration passing through his body like an electrical charge. I could feel the tension running out of his body. After about a half hour, I asked him to stand so that I could help with the alignment of his spine and the lengthening of his neck. I wanted to finish the session by making a slight adjustment to his neck. Because of his height, I stood on a chair behind him and gently lifted his head and neck. Meyer seemed very pleased with the session, and he graciously spread the word about my work. Within twenty-four hours, I was a very busy and popular addition to the team.

My next patient was a referral from the coach. Kenny had been hospitalized for dehydration. He had played hard the previous day and was not prepared for a difficult practice. It is not uncommon for players to become dehydrated; however, there are varying degrees of dehydration. His was severe, and his muscles had become contracted as a result of the dehydration. He was taken to the emergency room by ambulance and admitted as a patient.

I met Kenny when he was released from the hospital. He was eating fruit in an attempt to further hydrate himself. I was immediately impressed with Kenny's presence. He was only 6' 9", but he looked like a gigantic Ethiopian god. His arms were developed like honeydew melons and his thighs were like carved redwood tree trunks. He appeared uneasy and smiled a little shyly when he came to the door. His stutter was barely noticeable as he told me his story. He had been back from the hospital for only a few hours. His color was ashen, and he "just wanted a little energy."

I asked him if he had any other problems. He hesitated for a moment and then explained that just prior to this hospitalization he had his foot examined by a physician. He had had intense pain in that foot for nearly three years. He was told that he had a bone spur and arthritis in his foot.

I explained my procedure, being careful to emphasize that my touch is a very light one and that my fingers act to conduct the energy. He was open for the treatment and said that he had heard of people like me. I asked Kenny to lie diagonally on the bed. He was too tall to lie comfortably in any other position. I hopped onto the bed, seated myself in a cross-legged position, and touched his right hand.

As I allowed the energy to flow into his right wrist, Kenny relaxed. His breathing became regular and shallow. His eyelids started to flutter, and his body seemed to sink even further into the bed. He was in a trancelike state and remained in a state of deep relaxation for the next thirty minutes. During that time, I tried to increase the balance in his physical structure. I corrected the imbalances in the head and face, and drew energy down to Kenny's feet. I worked on his shoulders and his heart chakra (the area at his sternum). With gentle pressure, I aligned his hips. At the end of our session, I shook Kenny lightly. He started to blink his eyes and look around questioningly. "What did you do to me?" he asked. "I feel as if I can't move and weigh 300 pounds. I feel drugged."

I chuckled. What could I do with my 120 pounds that would knock out this larger-than-life creature? I explained to him that the healing energy has a relaxing effect and that his response was quite normal. Patients get very tired because of the intense internal cellular activity. I suggested that he take a nap and rest for the remainder of the day. He didn't argue. The man was barely capable of moving. This generally indicates a highly successful session.

The next day, when Kenny saw me, he was all smiles. Again he asked, "What did you do to me? I feel great." Kenny started practice again. He was still taking it easy and slowly building up to his normal training routine. He asked if we could meet for another session, and I very willingly obliged. We met in his room for his second treatment, but this time I asked him to sit upright in bed. We talked about everything and nothing. He told me that he was a musician. I told him that I too was a musician. He told me about his fifty-year-old girlfriend. I told him about my divorce and three children. During this mundane talk, I was working on his bone spur and patch of arthritis.

Suddenly, when I was touching his foot, I couldn't feel the bone spur or the patch of arthritis. I interrupted our conversation and told Kenny that I couldn't feel anything awry in his foot. I asked him to feel his foot, and he poked around and he could find nothing unusual. The two of us must have made an interesting sight looking for his lost patch of arthritis. I told Kenny that sometimes the energy will disperse arthritis in the course of healing other complaints, and apparently this is what happened. We were both elated. Kenny started to walk on his foot. He tried to move his foot in positions to create pain, but this was not possible.

After this dramatic episode, Kenny and I were moved to thank God for this blessed event. His friends picked us up at the motel, and we all went to an enthusiastic Baptist church, where we thanked God for this beautiful miracle.

Kenny wrote a very supportive letter in which he stated:

I'd like to thank you, Gloria. Without your help, I would not have made it through training. You are truly blessed by God.

Never before has anyone been able to help me with my feet. You not only helped me, but have made the arthritis go! Because of you, I'll be able to move like never before. The arthritis is gone. The spurs and calcium deposits have dissolved.

Kenny and I remained in contact with each other. He was eventually traded to a Turkish team. The last I heard from him was a call from Turkey. He wanted me to join his team—a tempting offer, though I couldn't see my way clear to leave California at that time.

Not all of the players were interested in hands-on-healing. Tom was a good case in point. He was an older, experienced player who had arthritis in his right knee. Trying to make a comeback, he took his training very seriously. Running across the court, he looked as if he were about to expire, but he never gave up. His knee was obviously a big problem for him. He favored his right leg and often limped after practice. I talked to him about my work, but he was not interested. He appreciated the fact that I did not persist in trying to talk him into trying a session.

Several days later, I talked to Tom about homeopathic remedies. He was still uninterested in a healing session but was willing to try something that he could ingest. I suggested a remedy that was a special combination for arthritis pain. We were able to get the remedy at a local health food store. The remedy was helpful, and after a short time, Tom started to get some relief. He started to have confidence in me and then allowed me to work on his knee. He was not up for a formal session, so I gently worked on his knee as we rode the bus to and from the gym. Tom was the coach's right-hand man and had a big influence on the team. His support was important, and I was happy to be able to help him. Although his knee improved, he decided not to play for the rest of the season. We talked about his decision, and he felt that this would be a good time to explore his spirituality and perhaps do some coaching with underprivileged children.

There were very few injuries during my time with the Cavs. The injuries were mainly the result of collisions. The players were extremely responsive to the yoga stretches and, consequently, were able to avoid serious injury. Meyer told a reporter from *The Oklahoman* that there were no injuries during this particular preseason practice other than those from collisions.

Danny was an energetic and wiry player. He was shorter than most of the players, but he was fast. During one practice, Danny collided with another player. We could hear the knees bounce off of each other—a foreboding sound. He was in intense pain. The trainer examined his knee and announced that he would have to be off of his feet for at least a week. We all felt terrible about this news. I offered to help, and I worked on him as we sat on the sidelines watching the practice. Focusing on the game, we were both somewhat unconscious of what was happening to his leg. Without too much effort on either one of our parts, Danny started to feel better. His knee became less swollen.

When we returned to the afternoon practice, the swelling had disappeared, and Danny wasn't feeling too much pain. I worked on the knee again, and by the end of practice, Danny was pain-free. The next day, he was re-examined by the trainer and given the OK to play. We were all delighted.

In Danny's note, he commented:

I can honestly say that the work and treatment of Dr. Kaye is very sufficient and dependable. I had a knee that was severely injured and due to the treatment, I can hereby say my knee has 95% recovered. I thank her and recommend her highly.

Another player who appreciated my work was Tony. He was an experienced, influential, former NBA player who had chronic stiffness in his back and was curious about the homeopathic remedies. I suggested a remedy specific to his condition. He began taking an over-the-counter homeopathic remedy called magnesium phosphate. Tony experienced almost immediate relief and generously shared his remedy with the rest of the team. It worked well on many of the players. The scene at the motel where we were all housed must have looked bizarre. The guys were passing remedies right and left.

"Hey, you got the mag phos?"

"No, Foster had it last."

"I thought Ron had it."

"No, Don had it the last time I saw it."

I was glad the remedies were welcomed, and I was tickled by the way they were passed around.

Tony had tight hamstrings. This was common among the players. He was very taken with the yoga classes and worked hard to increase his flexibility. I demonstrated positions that would help to increase mobility in particular areas.

On one occasion, Tony needed help getting up. I was the first person on the scene and literally lent a hand. Tony was seated with his back to the wall, and his legs were extended in front of him. I bent down and, facing him, put my hand on his forearm. I made a motion to help to propel him to a standing position, but it was to no avail. As it turned out, it took three of us to get Tony upright. He shook his lanky frame, got his sea legs, and went back to practice.

Most of the time, I was not conscious of the differences in our size, but with Tony and another player, Jawana, I was very conscious of my diminutive frame. Jawana had just come from a hair salon. He didn't want to be late, so he arrived at practice complete with deep conditioner on his hair and his cellular phone. I began to have a surrealistic feeling about life, limbs, hair conditioners, and cellular phones. He was the most astonishing looking player, over 7' tall, very thin, with endless legs. He was as flexible as a rubber band, and as he approached, he looked like a stalking flamingo right out of a Spielberg flick.

I was sitting on the sidelines, and he walked over to me. He said, "Could you stretch me out?" Not quite comprehending his request, I said, "Moi?" When he nodded to me, I had him lie on the floor. I assisted him as he moved one leg at a time. His first stretch consisted of lifting his leg to a ninety-degree angle. The second stretch called for more flexibility, creating a 120-degree angle. His flexibility and dedication to working his body certainly gained my admiration. Jawana's response to the training was gratifying, and he wrote the following note:

I have found great peace and an integration with my body and mind. Yoga has helped me concentrate more on mental awareness and controlling my body so that I may be 110% in my athletic workouts.

Gloria has helped my team overall with every aspect of training camp. Not only conditioning our bodies but our minds as well. Gloria has brought a new and profound aspect of training to the world of sports and fitness. She is highly respected by all who practice yoga including her coaches and staff.

As a farewell gesture, Meyer, Ray, and Don wanted to take me out for a night on the town. I was up for some two-stepping, but the cowboy bars in Oklahoma City did not appeal to the guys. We agreed on another bar that had a more neutral ambiance. I will never forget that cab ride. I sat in the back seat. Ray and Meyer got in with me, and I was completely overwhelmed by the impact of my escorts as they politely found places for their long legs and numerous elbows. I felt like a sardine in a packing plant.

When we arrived at the restaurant, heads turned. Tall basketball players and a short redhead made quite a showing. We had some drinks and some laughs. We all got a little teary-eyed. I hated to leave these guys. The day before, they joked with the newspaper reporter and told her that they were going to hide my plane ticket.

The next day, the coach drove me to the airport. I misread my departure time and missed my plane. I was forced to hang out in the airport lounge for a few hours. It was a good thing to do. It gave me time to reflect and prepare for re-entry into Santa Barbara.

My time with the Cavs was magical, and I was much enriched by the experience. It was such a leap for everyone concerned to have a healer in their midst.

More About Athletes

An Interview with Margaret

Margaret is a 5,000-meter runner and Olympic hopeful. Her approach to her training has become spiritual, and she meditates regularly. Her mission is to create national youth track programs.

Margaret: I was impressed with the results beginning with the first session. I tested the new changes in my body when I was running, and I was so happy with the results because my whole stride had changed. My center of gravity improved tremendously. Instead of running the way I was used to, striking with my heels in front of my body as if putting on the brakes, I was able to stride very fluidly and flowing. My legs, when they would strike the ground, would be perpendicular to the ground, giving me power and strength. It was very fluid, which makes a tremendous difference. As far as different changes in my body are concerned, from that first session my left leg had loosened up considerably, which allowed my hips to open up, making my body feel more balanced and stable. During the second session, which was just two days ago, we had worked on overall body changes, and I felt my balance improve considerably.

Dr. Kaye: Could you comment on your Olympic aspirations and determination? When I viewed your videos, I was so impressed with your ability. I understand you will be training with a coach in New Zealand who works with Olympic athletes. Could you tell me about your dream?

Margaret: I am very excited. Next month I will be traveling to New Zealand, where I'll train with Arthur Lydiard. I have always wanted to be an Olympic runner. Running is an activity I've loved for a long, long time. I started competing in the seventh grade, and I've thrived on the time spent training. I like to compete and challenge myself and really see the best in myself come out. I have enjoyed many friendships connected with my training and am most relaxed and comfortable when I am out on the track. I am very dedicated and determined to develop my ability. I feel that I have a lot more ability and am working on having that come out. I can visualize where I want to be, and I feel like I'm free and flying along effortlessly. When I run, I see how fluid ballet dancers can be. I know that is where I want to be. I know that is where I am headed. During the last week, I could feel that I am getting closer to that goal and it will be possible for me to achieve that goal.

Dr. Kaye: It has been a tremendous joy for me to work with you. Your sensitivity just speaks to everything that we have been doing. You have been very responsive. During our second session, I worked on an imbalance in your rib cage. I'd like you to describe the results as well as the work we did with your feet.

Margaret: That session was incredible. The most prominent difference occurred after you worked on the right side of my rib cage. There was a lot of tension that was stored up in there, and after five or ten minutes it was completely gone. I was able to relax that area. It opened up my whole rib cage, and also my right leg became more stable. I appreciated learning exercises for my feet and toes. I had never considered the importance of them, but after doing a few exercises I realized that I am more stable, strong, and balanced. It was very exciting to feel what a balanced body feels like.

Dr. Kaye: Margaret, could you tell me what other modalities you have tried in order to reach this kind of fluidity?

Margaret: One thing that I felt was helping me was tai chi. I felt that there was a lot of fluidity while doing these stretches, but it was more of a chore than something that I really wanted to do. I went through ten sessions of a Rolfing process. Through deep massage, I was able to feel more balanced and I was able to release emotions that were built up since childhood. It was very helpful.

Dr. Kaye: Could you compare the work that we have done with the other treatments?

Margaret: There were definite results from the Rolfing. They were not always noticeable at first, and it would take much longer to achieve those results. The emotional purging was very difficult at times. It was also painful when muscles would not want to let go. There was usually an emotion caught up with that, and I would walk around with that until my next session, and eventually it would let go. The results that I achieved in a week with you have been almost instantaneous. The healing session is incredible. I don't know how it happens, but it happens without anything I have to try to do. It just does it by itself. I don't have to think. I don't have to be conscious, and I don't have to go back to those childhood experiences to piece a puzzle together. It works.

Dr. Kaye: We just completed our third session, and we worked on your neck. That was something that needed attention. We also worked a little more on the hips and pelvis. Would you like to comment on today's session?

Margaret: I was looking forward to seeing if I could make some improvements with my neck. My neck felt very stiff and compact before I came in. Now, I feel that my neck is an extension of my spine. It is lifting me up. The muscles have relaxed and are now very, very soft. The flexibility that I have is just incredible, and I am now able to move my neck in ways that were impossible before coming here. My body feels incredible right now.

As far as the pelvis area is concerned, it is starting to become more my natural posture than trying to think about it as before. It is just starting to feel more comfortable the way it is.

Dr. Kaye: Do you have a final comment? Any advice to people about this type of treatment?

Margaret: It definitely works. People would be so fortunate to have Gloria working on and with them. It has made a tremendous difference for me.

An Interview with Yulia

Yulia is a dancer; I met her when I was taking classes with her. After a short time, Yulia talked to me about her rheumatoid arthritis. She shared her experience through a conversational interview.

Yulia: I was devastated; besides the pain in my back, I could feel that the inflammation was going into my wrists and other parts of my body. After the first session, I felt a warmth in my back and a release…I felt like I was on the right track.

Dr. Kaye: So, you were feeling the rheumatoid arthritis throughout your body?

Yulia: I could feel the progression of the condition. If you have something that keeps prevailing, it is a very devastating feeling…it's something you cannot stop. So, I was very concerned at that time.

Dr. Kaye: You have a strong history of competing with your dance, and your expertise has been acknowledged in many ways; were you concerned about your future as a dancer?

Yulia: Yes, I was. I was starting to get a little bit depressed, to say the least! Dance is my breath; it's such a part of my being; it's my purpose!

Dr. Kaye: Your purpose. And, getting back to your body, you were identified with rheumatoid arthritis through laboratory tests? And most recently you have been tested again, and there was no evidence of the rheumatoid arthritis, clinically?

Yulia: Yes, that was actually quite a shocking fact—I mean, a *good* shocking fact!—that the tests indicated that there was no evidence of rheumatoid arthritis.

Dr. Kaye: So, you must be very happy now—dancing more freely, knowing that you have a future, and that the rheumatoid arthritis is history for you.

Yulia: Yes, it relieves a lot of pressure knowing that something is not going to eat you up! It liberates so much more energy for me to focus on my dancing and not be afraid of what's going to happen to me.

Dr. Kaye: Very good. Thank you.

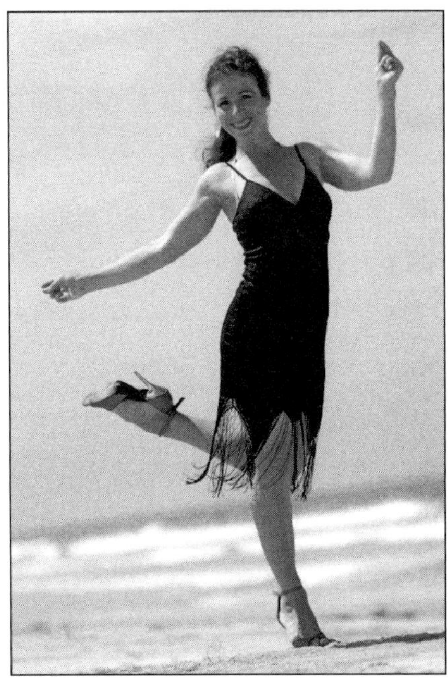

Yulia

An Interview with John

John is a musician, piano tuner, and father of three young children. He is athletic, and his back pain used to interfere with his basketball practice. Now, he feels like a kid again and gets out on the court regularly.

John: I have had a lot of pain in the sacrum and the back of my spine. The pain worked itself up to the middle of my back and then moved into my neck and shoulders.

Dr. Kaye: When did you first begin to have problems?

John: Severe, noticeable pain started about twelve years ago.

Dr. Kaye: What have you tried to do to correct your problems?

John: I went to chiropractors primarily, and I was diagnosed as having a shorter leg. I have seen three chiropractors and have been treated by them. The results were not very encouraging. My pain shifted, and I had pain in new areas. I continued with this treatment because I was of the belief that if the body changed and the spine shifted, I would naturally feel pain.

Dr. Kaye: And then you decided to have a healing session?

John: Yes.

Dr. Kaye: What was your experience with that?

John: I had immediate results. I had no pain; I took the insert out of my shoe and immediately started walking. It was the first time in ten years that I felt I could just walk without thinking 'this hurts', or 'I have to watch out for that.'

Dr. Kaye: So you had a sense of freedom about your body?

John: Yes. It felt the way it was when I was a kid. I didn't have to think about what I was doing. I had been used to watching everything carefully, and now I find myself walking without my lift and feeling no pain.

Dr. Kaye: Do you remember what the treatment felt like?

John: It was primarily relaxing. It felt warm, and I had sensations of energy shooting throughout my body. I felt a gradual shifting of my weight. Tension was released, and a gradual balancing action was happening.

Dr. Kaye: Would you say that after your healing session your pain level decreased?

John: The pain totally went away. All of the leg, spine, and back pain went away. The only funny thing was my left shoulder. It had a few kinks in it, but then that went away as well. It felt like my body was shifting.

Dr. Kaye: Your back, then, has been much more comfortable. Have your sinuses also improved?

John: My back is very comfortable, and my sinuses feel shifted. The congestion itself seems to have gone away.

Dr. Kaye: What finally convinced you to do a session?

John: I had a severe cold and tried homeopathy and the chiropractor again. Nothing was working, so out of instinct, I decided to give this a try. This may sound kind of corny, but I think it was God's way of getting me to move along my path.

Dr. Kaye: Could you talk about your experience?

John: I have done a lot of things, and it is always great to get results. That is what one hopes for. After a while, one gets used to disappointment and accepts the limitations of the various treatment modalities. I was really surprised that our session worked the first time. I have tried acupuncture and you name it, and none of the treatments have worked so immediately and completely. The thing about this healing is that it takes into account the whole picture. I tell my wife all the time that I would just as soon be saved by Grace as by work. I would much rather do it that way…have God do it.

Dr. Kaye: Do you feel God's presence?

John: Absolutely. I do not think it would work without God. To me, it is unexplainable, but I have come to realize that most things are unexplainable anyway.

Dr. Kaye: Is there anything you would like to add?

John: I would like to comment on the process itself. It had a lot more impact than I expected, and in the course of doing it, I really felt more than I would have dreamed. Today in particular, I was kind of overwhelmed. I was just sitting on the chair; you were working on my back, and I began to feel like I was getting knocked out…I felt like I was going to conk out. I came in here with plenty of energy, and I have plenty of energy now. However, at the time, I felt like I was about to keel over. Where is the bed?

Dr. Kaye: My explanation for that is that so much internal activity is occurring that it becomes very tiring. On a cellular level, so much is going on. Scientists have commented that cells become rearranged through this process and that the process accelerates the regeneration of cells.

John: From my results, I believe, this is exactly what happens.

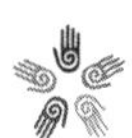

C h a p t e r   7

Progress With Forward-Thinking Physicians

My commitment to work with the medical community is ongoing, and I have always seen myself working side-by-side with the physician. My experience with physicians has been varied. I have been embraced by some and tolerated or rejected by others. In the early seventies, I was laughed at by a group of physicians when I spoke about my use of yoga as a treatment modality with heroin addicts. In the late seventies, when I was the principle investigator for a large government-funded research project that studied the effects of yoga on substance abusers, there was no laughter. There was inquisitiveness, support, and the beginnings of a blending of various disciplines.

One of my more supportive experiences has been working with Rodney Paragas, M.D., a warm, open, caring being. He has been a great source of comfort to me and many of my clients. I met Rod in

September of 1988. I was doing one of my many fasts and arrived at his office with freshly juiced apples. The thick, slightly green juice had the look of a sick urine sample. We sat in his very non-medical office with this big bottle between us. When I explained that this was not a urine sample but rather freshly juiced apples, he readily agreed to partake in this noxious-looking delicacy.

Sipping this fluid in long-stemmed wine glasses, we began our professional relationship. At the time, I was interested in meeting physicians who could provide holistic health care at my center for elders. Rod formerly had a huge family practice in Central California and was eminently qualified to assist me at my center.

One of the first elderly patients he treated was a woman resident who had been released from the hospital even though she was actively having a stroke. Although it was after hours, I called Rod. He confirmed my suspicions and reassured me at the same time. This was so typical of the many interactions we have had over the years. His willingness to participate, listen, and hear with all of his being immediately sets him apart from so many others. I appreciate appropriate medical backup, and Rod has always been there for me in a non-intrusive, supportive way.

His practice of energetic medicine attracts the seekers. His father was "an old country doctor" from Nebraska. Rod takes his time with patients, maintaining the tradition established by his father. His unwillingness to buy into the system prompted him to come to California to seek additional exposure in alternative medicine. He sees "…alternative medicine as a better way of treating people."

When Rod finally settled in California and associated with a clinic in San Luis Obispo, he offered options to his patients. "When people came in with pain, I offered them alternatives. Some of them took it, and some of them didn't. The patients that did, improved. That solidified my interest and gave me the feedback that I needed to prove to me that it was a legitimate type of medicine even in the seventies."

Rod and I collaborated on a number of cases. Our mutual patients have included ones with cancer, resistant pain, digestive complaints, anxiety, and depression. Our collaborations have been supportive with each of us bringing our knowledge, intuition, and expertise to the patient. Commenting on healers, Rod says, "We have evidence now that spiritual healing, or laying on of hands, not only positively affects the energetic body but the physiology of the living system." Rod believes that alternative medicine is becoming more acceptable. He adds, "I see that trend continuing with the government being more interested in developing protocols to understand alternative medicine, energetic medicine, and acupuncture. Medical schools are now teaching and requiring students to learn how to communicate and listen to their patients. There is a move to getting back to establishing rapport with the patient."

Cynthia Mervis-Watson, M.D., Long-Time Supporter and Friend

"For years, I have had the good fortune to practice what I love, medicine. One of the first things I learned was to be very present with patients and to listen. Oftentimes people want to be heard and not judged. I have tried to focus on reflecting love and acceptance. From years of listening to patients, I have found that emotional trauma underlies most physical illness. These issues need to be addressed in order to help the patient get well. I have been surprised that people have felt better even when, technically, I didn't "do" anything. Just being present with them and allowing them to express their emotions, fears and anxieties can have a profound effect.

The healing process requires regeneration, and this is where the healer has an essential role. The healer can help patients recreate balance by supplying them with love and healing energy until they can generate it on their own. Rarely does the doctor learn anything about this aspect of healing. Patients need to be surrounded with practitioners who can give them love and attention. Doctors seldom have the time, patience or even the understanding of how this process works. Too often I hear patients complain that doctors won't even answer questions let alone give them an encouraging word. It makes me sad for my profession.

I will often recommend that a patient learn to meditate or see a healer. Various techniques will work for different people. We have different belief systems that make a difference in how each of us responds to various therapies. You have to treat the patient within the structure of his or her own belief system. I have patients who will do well with natural therapies and others who won't.

In the future, I see physicians, healers and other alternative health practitioners working together to encourage healing in a new and more effective way."

—Cynthia Mervis Watson, M.D.

Daisy Green, Osteopathic Physician

Daisy Green, D.O., is an osteopathic physician who grew up in Kansas. She has a large practice and works twelve-hour days. She is loved by her patients and spends a full hour with each one of them.

Her treatment rooms look into her garden, and a feeling of serenity and tranquility pervade the setting. She is a meditator and hopes to create an interdisciplinary setting in which massage, healing, acupuncture, yoga, aromatherapy, and osteopathy can blend.

Daisy requested that we meet after she heard that I was successfully doing long-distance healing on one of her teenage patients who had pronounced scoliosis. The teenager rejected medical help and was in complete denial regarding her deformity.

We connected immediately, and I was impressed with her low-key demeanor. Daisy had never planned on being a physician. "I didn't like physicians. I thought physicians were arrogant and cruel," she stated. Her brother-in-law, who is a doctor of osteopathy, influenced her decision to pursue a medical degree. She had been a research microbiologist and found that the isolation associated with research did not suit her. She told me about some of the stresses involved in trying to create an interdisciplinary center.

I demonstrated my techniques. Daisy was a very willing subject and, after experiencing the effects of the healing, suggested that we meet for more sessions. At the end of our third session, Daisy commented on the future of the medical profession and a greater acceptance of alternative medicine. She asserts:

I don't believe that you can suppress forever the innate knowledge that we have. It has only been in the past few hundred years that we have had this crazy idea that we can take the body in and of itself and treat certain parts and that's that. For most of our history we have believed in an integrated approach to healing. We have respected how important it is for the person to heal themselves.

Daisy believes that healers and physicians can work together. She suggests that healers align themselves with physicians who are accepting of healers and, as that becomes a well-established and accepted team that has good trust in the community, then what becomes available is the next level of physician who might be more curious than the established, more orthodox physician. She has positive thoughts for the future and believes that alternative methods of healing slowly and quietly will be considered by many more physicians.

Michael Stulberg, M.D., Psychiatrist

Dr. Michael Stulberg is a caring, attentive psychiatrist who exudes a very empathic attitude. He is a friend and a source of tremendous support.

Dr. Stulberg: I am a psychiatrist. Since 1976, I have been in private practice and am the medical director of a chemical dependency unit at what used to be Pinecrest Hospital. Pinecrest is now known as Cottage Care Center. I am a board-certified psychiatrist having been trained in psychiatry and child psychiatry at the University of Michigan.

Some years ago, you conducted relaxation training groups on the chemical dependency unit. Every once in a while a patient out of that group would talk with you or request your help with some type of a physical problem—whether it was headaches, backaches, anxiety, or some kind of pain problem. They would get back to me and report that they felt better. Whatever you did worked and worked fairly miraculously. They frequently asked if they could continue to see you for treatment for whatever the problem was. I began to think that something was going on here. We went out to lunch several times and you explained what it is that you do. Patients were telling me that whatever you were doing was working when other things hadn't helped. I was impressed.

Dr. Kaye: I remember working on many physical complaints that accompanied substance abuse—injuries from automobile accidents, digestive complaints, headaches. These complaints are not necessarily associated with substance abuse but seem to arise from a lifestyle in which people are not really conscious about their health.

Dr. Stulberg: I would like to mention that you were working with a group of people who are fairly hard-boiled, hard-nosed, and are not particularly into health. These people would normally be very suspicious of a self-care approach. But, in spite of that population, they took to you, they liked you, and they believed in you. They really enjoyed the groups. It wasn't that you just got results with particular problems but you also won over a population that is not very easy to win over.

Dr. Kaye: I know that the energy can be a very strong force and with the relaxation that can accompany this infusion of energy, defensive behavior can be diminished.

Dr. Stulberg: I have an idea how it happens on a much more super-ficial level. In my work in the chemical dependency field, I have found that the one quality people must have to work in the field is genuineness. You can't be putting on something that you aren't to people who are alcoholics and drug addicts. You have to be whoever you really are whether that is a physician or a counselor in the field. I think that genuineness is a characteristic of people who work in the chemical dependency field. I think that is absolutely necessary, and, without that, you cannot have relationships with people. They can smell falsehood.

Dr. Kaye: Could you comment on physicians in general and their reluctance to look at alternative forms of treatment?

Dr. Stulberg: Physicians in the West are grounded in Western medicine. Physicians in the East are grounded in Eastern medicine. What you do is more grounded in Eastern medicine. Shifting of energies is more of an Eastern concept. I think there is a real reluctance on the part of Western physicians to accept and understand and work with an approach to the body which is not Western in its basic origin. The idea of energies, blocked energies, and imbalances as a solution to a specific problem, or to a specific organ, is something that doesn't make a lot of sense to someone who is trained in Western medicine. There are inroads and forays into alternative medicine that are probably more prevalent than ever before. The bottom line, I think, for anyone, whether they are trained Eastern or Western, is if something works, that's terrific.

For myself, I don't think I am particularly open-minded in terms of my ability to learn new things or implement new things in my own practice, but I try to be open-minded in terms of ideologies. Nobody has a corner on the truth, and even though I'm not familiar with the basis of the techniques that you use and even though I don't understand in a Western sense how it works, I am practical, and if something works, then I am going to stick with it.

Star Trek Medicine: Progressive Times

In August of 1994, I had the pleasure of lecturing at the University of Miami's medical school. The medical school developed a comprehensive pain clinic that had state-of-the-art equipment and a holistic approach to pain resolution. A team approach dominated the program and a family atmosphere was created by this dedicated crew. Patients were kept active throughout the day. Meals were served in a dormitory fashion, and the patients' families also became part of the treatment protocol.

I addressed approximately fifty medical personnel, which included physicians, nurses, and occupational and physical therapists. My good friend, Pat Pier, R.N., arranged for my talk and introduced me to this prestigious group. For the most part, this adventurous group was open to my presentation. There were a few skeptics and about five people left as soon as it was courteous to do so.

Many variations of the techniques that I demonstrated were already being used at the clinic. For example, meditation and relaxation techniques were part of the program. One nurse commented, "When you go within yourself and take time each day to go within, you rejuvenate the physical, mental, and the whole bit."

When I demonstrated techniques for bringing energy to the hands, nearly everyone who participated was able to experience a magnetic force field between their hands. At the end of the lecture, there were many questions about the application of these techniques.

I visited the hospital for several more days and saw that I had made significant connections with the group. One nurse brought her aging mother to see me about her digestive and arthritic complaints. Another nurse sought my services for a pre-operative energy boost, and a staff physician consulted me regarding homeopathic cell salts. My visit to Miami reinforced my desire to associate with a medical school. Exposure to alternative methods will be important for the blending of traditional and alternative health care. I have even had the honor and pleasure of lecturing at UCLA School of Medicine.

I have treated many physicians and nurses. It is always a delight to watch their healing process. One nurse, who worked for an orthopedic surgeon, consulted me about her painful bone spur. After her first visit, she was surprised to be able to walk without pain. We continued to see each other for several more visits and were able to watch the deformity in her foot disappear. Another nurse elected to have spinal fusion and my work with her rapidly reduced healing time. An emergency room nurse experienced a lingering sinus infection. After exhausting all possible medical interventions, we did some significant healing work, and her sinus condition was relieved.

Overall, I have incredible respect and compassion for physicians. My compassion and understanding extends to the misinformed and closed-minded. There was a time when I had no compassion for the dedicated, hard-working, poorly informed physician, and then it dawned on me that it is ludicrous to condemn or judge. I look at my enlightened physician friends and in some ways their struggle is even more intense than mine. As physicians, they do battle for significant changes in medical practice and attempt to educate the public as well as traditional physicians. They work from within the system to effect change.

The profession seems to be slowly changing. It is no longer the exclusive, prestigious, ivory tower male-dominated community. There are widening cracks in the fortress.

The world of health care is rapidly changing. Americans are demanding positive, effective interventions. Healers are beginning to receive the recognition they deserve. Many are surprised when I indicate the number of physicians who are supportive of my work. Health care is evolving as never before, and we are blessed to be riding this wave. The challenge has changed, as has the nature of the work. I no longer justify what I do. I just do it.

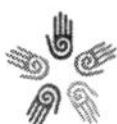

SECTION II
Healing Basics and Insights

Chapter 8

Healing for Beginners

Introduction

I have treated everything from bellyaches, heartaches, backaches, spider bites, migraines, bunions, and everything in between. Most of the time I forget how extraordinary the healing process is. I expect positive change, and more than 90 percent of the time this is achieved. The energy immediately addresses the distress and change occurs. The energy assists the body into wellness. Whether it is something as simple as bringing an embedded splinter to the surface of the skin or a more serious condition such as reducing a cancerous tumor, healing aids the body as it naturally wants to be healthy and whole.

The medical community calls on me more and more, and I have now trained a number of physicians in the healing process. I am frequently challenged by individuals who have the preconceived notion that this process cannot be taught. I am able to teach about 40 percent of what I do to interested parties. This becomes a self-selecting group; gifted or sensitive people are usually those who have this interest.

For the first time, I have presented a detailed description of the process. As of this writing I am of the belief that this process affects the body cellularly. According to my notion, cells are dispersed, reorganized, or regenerated.

For example, in the case of arthritis, unwanted cells are dispersed and many arthritic conditions begin to immediately resolve. When cells regenerate, the area around an incision can appear healthier. Black and blue marks begin to fade. Wounds begin to heal. In a twenty-four-hour period, the open ulcer on a diabetic foot improved 50 percent. Again, these are examples of rapid cellular transformation.

The photograph below is of a diabetic ulcer. An open ulcerated wound is frequently seen in diabetic patients. Traditional medical treatment was ineffective with this condition. After one treatment and a time lapse of twenty-four hours, the size of the ulcer reduced about 50 percent. The ulcer healed from the underside of the foot and regenerated new skin. The white space you see between the two sores in the right photo is skin that was regenerated overnight.

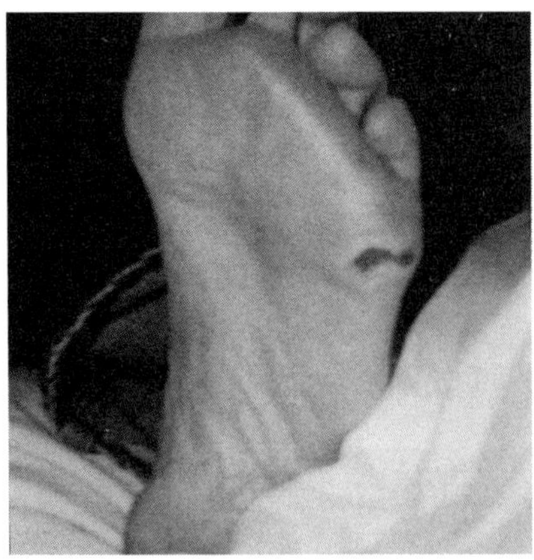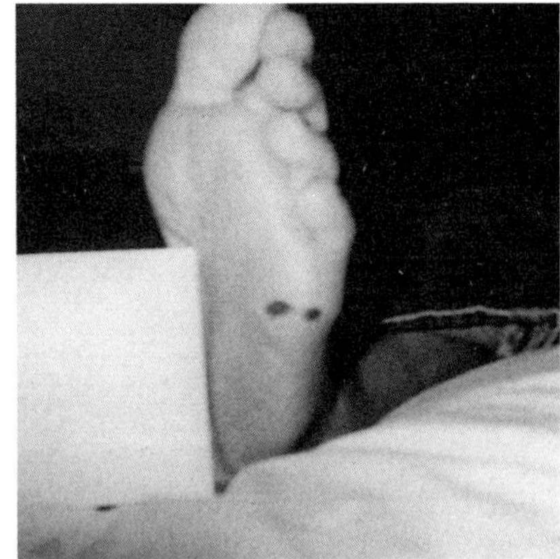

When cells reorganize, many complaints of pain reduce. Back pain, whether it is chronic or acute, is usually affected by this reorganization. As the muscles and ligaments release, the structure becomes more aligned. The more balanced the body, the less pain one experiences.

The techniques I describe are rather straightforward. Basically, these techniques help to create balance in the body. Due to the fact that the energy is far more intelligent than we are, it will go to where it is needed. These techniques will enable you to assist the body into a greater state of health.

This information may be used by anyone who has an interest in helping to heal the angst of this planet. The healing energy addresses the physical, emotional, and spiritual aspects of life. As a practitioner you are also nourished by the energy.

Some may use this information in a professional practice. The techniques have no unpleasant side effects; however if you do not see immediate change with someone who is very ill, consult medical personnel. This is not just meant to be a disclaimer. These techniques are offered to assist in a healing interaction.

How to Begin

Please follow the instructions carefully. These techniques are subtle, and at first you might feel as if you are not experiencing the energetic effects. Have patience and you will soon become sensitive to these subtleties. A light touch is usually more effective than a heavier touch. As you apply these techniques to friends, family, and clients, you will probably be pleasantly surprised by the results.

I believe that the interested student can learn how to use these techniques. Whether the student becomes the healer or not is another consideration. Everyone can draw a line, but not everyone is an artist. The degree to which one becomes committed to the application of these techniques is a determining factor. Relax and enjoy the world of healing.

Creating Healing Hands

The following exercise is intended to generate healing energy in the hands. Sit in a comfortable position. Place your hands on your thighs and, with your palms up, take several deep breaths. Begin to relax. Gently lift your hands about one-half inch from your thighs. From this point all of your movements will appear to be involuntary. Your hands will move at an imperceptible rate. When your hands are chest-high allow your fingertips to face each other. There will be a magnetic force radiating from your fingertips. With the energy moving through your fingertips you will feel as if there is a ball of energy between your hands. Slowly move that energy up to your face. Gently touch your face with the energy you have created in your hands. With the same slow intention allow your hands to return to your thighs. Be very gentle with yourself as you resume an ordinary consciousness.

You will probably find it helpful to read the following script into a tape recorder. The total time for this exercise is five to ten minutes.

1. Sit in a comfortable chair and place your hands on your thighs (pause for fifteen seconds).

2. Take several deep breaths (pause for sixty seconds).

3. Allow your hands to gently move from the thighs (pause for two minutes).

4. Allow fingertips to point toward each other (pause for thirty seconds).

5. Experience the energy between your hands (pause for one minute).

6. Raise your hands to your face and gently touch your face (pause for one minute).

7. Slowly lower your hands (pause for two minutes).

Remain still as the more ordinary consciousness returns to you. This is a very powerful exercise, and having once experienced the energy in the hands it is very difficult to dispute the existence of this phenomenon.

Application of Energy

Assessing and Treating Imbalances in the Face

Now that you have experienced this energy, the next step is to learn when, how, and where to place your hands. To do this, you need to assess the imbalances in the body. Students are usually bewildered when I talk about structural imbalances; however, within a short time these subtle imbalances become visible to the newly trained eye. This exercise requires a partner.

Sit in front of your partner and very carefully examine your partner's face.

Begin at the forehead.

Are the planes of the forehead similar?

Does one side protrude more than the other side?

How similar in character are both sides of the forehead?

Make a mental note about the imbalance.

Move to the eyebrows.

Are the arches of the eyebrows different?

Does this difference relate to the planes in the forehead?

Carefully look at the character of the eyes.

Is one livelier than the other?

Ask your partner to gaze at an area above your head that is about twenty feet away. When the partner is gazing in this manner, do the eyes look equally focused? Sometimes the difference in the gaze is related to the angling in the forehead, and at other times eyestrain can account for this difference.

Look at the angling of the cheekbones.

Does one seem higher than the other?

Are the cheeks similar?

Is the angling of the jaw similar?

How is the head placed on the neck?

This is an exercise in seeing. Many students are astonished that they can easily see once they know how and where to look. Now where are we going to place the hands? It's natural to want to go to the main area of distress. Consider this possibility, however. The main area of distress is probably deficient, and this deficiency may contribute to distress. The side of the body opposite the distress usually holds an over-energy. By placing the hands on the side that has the over-energy you are encouraging the energy to move to the deficient side. This has nothing to do with trigger points, acupressure points, massage, Reiki, etc. This has to do with the logical distribution of energy. I believe that one of the reasons my clients frequently experience immediate change has to do with distribution of energy. How does the energy make structural changes? I don't believe that the energy makes the structural change, but rather the energy releases the muscles and ligaments that are improperly holding the structure. This system relaxes the muscles and allows the structure of the body to be more symmetrical. The more symmetrical the body, the more the energy efficiently moves through the body, including moving into the areas of distress.

Once again, look at your partner. The placement of the hands is as important as the intention of the student. This is not a massage technique, and the hands need to be held in a still, reverent manner. I'm not suggesting that there be formal prayer before placing the hands or that the student have a serious pious attitude. I am suggesting that the student have an intention to serve as a conduit for energy. The correction will be made with the infusion of energy and the body will naturally move into balance. Energy makes the corrections in a manner similar to water seeking its own level. A light to moderate sustained touch rather than a stroking motion allows the energy to be communicated with greater ease. The face may reflect other imbalances in the body. Disturbances in the face can be an indication of back pain, neck pain, and gastrointestinal distress.

Assessing and Treating Imbalances in the Neck

Structural imbalances in the neck can create a wide variety of complaints. Imbalances must be assessed before they can be corrected. Just as we carefully looked at the imbalances in the face, we will now slowly make our assessments of the neck. Sit across from your partner. Ask your partner to look directly above the top of your head. Ask your partner to soften the gaze and relax.

Look very carefully at the placement of the head on the neck.

Does it appear that the head is skewed to one side?

Is the jaw line significantly different on each side?

How similar is the space between the ear and the shoulder?

Sit to the side of your partner so that you get a good view of the way the head is carried.

Does your partner lead with the head?

Is there an unwanted hump at the base of the neck?

Could you be looking at a straight "military" type neck?

Sit at the back of your partner's neck.

What are you seeing?

Is there a tightness or more of a resistance on one side than the other?

Are you attracted to any particular areas of the neck?

At this point you will frequently hear comments from your partner as to where the aches might be. Please do not be intimidated or influenced by what you are told. Use the information and then test the theory that the side opposite the area of complaint is the one that actually needs the attention. There is usually an area of over-energy on the side opposite the complaint area. By placing your hands on the over-energy you are actually helping to distribute and move the energy to the area of deficit.

Of course, there are always exceptions to this basic principle. Still, reread the instructions for balancing the energy of the face and see if the instructions come together for you. Check to see how the base of the skull is placed on the neck. Do you see imbalances? I usually like to make corrections in this area using my thumbs. Place slightly more pressure on the side of the neck that has more resistance to the touch. This is usually the side where there is less complaint. By working on the neck you will be able to assist with releasing sinus pressure, headaches, eyestrain, sore throats, and the obvious neck pain.

Neck Adjustment

I like to make a neck adjustment using a gentle pressure. Stand behind your partner. Have your partner stand upright with feet parallel to each other and with the hands at the sides bisecting the thighs. Have your partner lock the knees and tighten the buttocks. Place your index fingers on the jaw and gently lift the head. This action lengthens the spine. I like the person receiving the treatment to close their eyes, and with eyes closed roll the eyes upward.

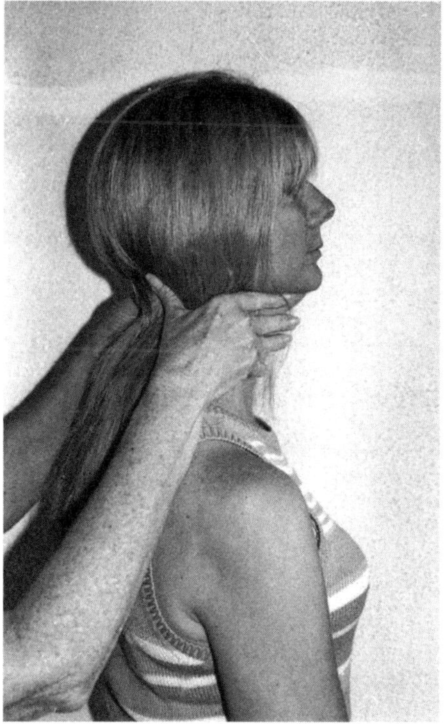

Neck Adjustment

With each adjustment have the client roll the eyes upward and then relax, and let a normal gaze return to the client. This is a very powerful, yet simple exercise. I recommend making this adjustment three times before asking if any change has occurred. After you have manipulated the neck three consecutive times allow the client to rest. Frequently the client will feel lightheaded because of the amount of energy moving through the body. Try to spot your client by lightly touching the arm. This gesture will let your client know that you are available for physical support.

Assessing and Treating Imbalances in the Back

Have your partner stand directly in front of you. Look at the angle of the shoulders.

Is one higher than the other?

Is the character of the shoulder different?

Does one come farther forward than the other?

Now look at the character of the shoulder blades.

Is one higher than the other one?

Does one seem more pronounced than the other?

Is one shoulder blade coming forward?

Move to the spine; run your fingers along either side of the spine.

Can you feel a greater definition on one side?

Is there a thickening on one side that is not present on the other?

Move to the mid-back.

Do the muscles below the shoulder blades seem equally balanced?

Is the area above the shoulder blades more concave on one side than the other?

Look at the hips.

Is one hip higher than the other one?

Is one hip more forward than the other?

Do the right and left buttocks have a similar character?

Does one seem more toned than the other?

Can you see areas of deficit in the buttocks?

These are some basic questions you can ask yourself when you are assessing imbalances in the back. The entire assessment takes less than a minute. As your intuition becomes more finely honed, you will quickly go to the areas of deficit and have a better sense of the possible ways of correcting the deficits.

Balancing the Chakras

The notion of the chakras comes from an ancient Hindu tradition. The word is pronounced "shock-rah," and although it is part of the new age lingo there is nothing new about the chakras. The chakras are a construct, which means that they are ideas rather than something tangible that can be excised or palpated.

This technique of balancing the chakras was originally shown to me by Richard Moss, M.D. He was shown the technique by Brough Joy, M.D., who in turn was taught by a layperson. I have modified the original presentation, which Richard called "sacred meditation." I found this technique to be rather straightforward, and it is a very good way to experience an energy and apply it in a systematic way. It also is excellent for dealing with an immune system dysfunction. The chakras loosely correlate to the endocrine system. Theoretically, when the chakras are balanced the endocrine system will function more efficiently. The functioning of the endocrine system influences the functioning of the immune system. This technique is very useful for enhancing and activating a powerful energy flow. It is useful in helping to resolve painful injuries, headaches, and sinus conditions. It also seems to help with circulatory problems.

Instructions for Balancing the Energy of the Chakras

Please record the following instructions:

Have your partner lie down. Hold your partner's right wrist with your right hand. Hold the wrist with the intention of assisting the body into a relaxed state. Move your hand palm down, from the pelvis to over the top of your partner's head. Repeat this motion three to six times. Move slowly over the body and make sure that your hand is three to four inches above the physical body. Place your hand over the area between the breasts. The heart chakra is located about midpoint on the sternum. This loosely correlates to the thymus. Production of T-cells is attributed to the thymus, and so this area is of particular importance in treating diseases of the immune system. Let your hand hover over this area until you feel a gentle vibration. If it is difficult to feel any sensation, move your hand in a slow clockwise rotation and see if that stimulates sensation. You can also make spider-like movements with your hands, or if you still feel no activity, place your index finger on the midpoint of the sternum and apply a gentle pressure to this area. Hopefully, you will now have experienced a sensation under your finger. If this is not the case, not to worry; this is just the very beginning of this exercise.

Now let's go to the throat chakra. Again, activate this area by holding your hands three to five inches from the throat. This area roughly correlates to the thyroid. Now move to the solar plexus and allow your hand to hover over this area. Maintain this position for up to a full minute. The third eye, or the area between the eyebrows, correlates to the pituitary gland. It is also considered to be the witnessing chakra. This chakra allows us to witness life with a sense of healthy detachment. Individuals who have sinus problems, or particular difficulties with vision, may have a stubborn resistance in this area. The area should be soft and pliable. The next area to be activated is about two inches from the southernmost tip of the pelvis. This area is a very telling one. In the United States, this area is frequently over-energized. However, if there are extenuating circumstances such as infection, cancer, or low libidinal energy, this area may be somewhat dulled. If I find a need to specifically stimulate this area, I always ask permission to touch this potentially sensitive area. When permission is given to stimulate this area, apply a moderate pressure to the slight indentation about two inches from the end of the pelvis.

The top of the head is next to be activated. Try to find the area midpoint in the skull. This is the point that would be the soft spot for a baby. It is said that very evolved yogis actually have a soft spot at the top of the head that is similar to a baby's. The soft spot is created by the energy moving through the body. Individuals with headaches and neurological symptoms frequently have very resistant areas in the head. To stimulate this area, gently touch the top of the head with the index finger and make a small, slow, clockwise rotation with the finger. When you are finished with this gentle massage, hold your hand above the top of the head and try to make contact with the energy coming from the top of the head. Pull this energy upward by moving your hand about five inches from the top of the head. When this is completed, go to the feet.

Place your hand so that the balls of the feet are facing the palms of your hands. Your fingertips are pointed toward the heels. Pull the energy by moving the hands six to eight inches from the feet and then returning to the original position. This will manipulate and strengthen the energy moving through the body. Maintain this position for thirty to sixty seconds. Move to the head and begin to reverse your movement. Move to the feet. Place your hand over the third eye. Move to the pelvis. Place your hand above the throat. Move to the heart chakra. Once again, to close the exercise sit next to your partner, place your hand three inches above the pelvis and make a sweeping gesture from the pelvis to the top of the head. After repeating this movement four to six times, sit quietly next to your partner and place your hand gently on your partner's right wrist. Have a quiet moment with your partner.

Long-Distance Healing

The system of long-distance healing that I use is something that I've developed over the years. Years ago, my friend telephoned me and asked me to heal her sore throat. I had never done a long-distance healing before and I wasn't quite sure where to begin. As I mentioned in Chapter 1, I had met healer Barbara Ivanova during my trip to Russia. She never actually showed me her long-distance healing technique, but from my experience with her I learned about possibilities.

As I listened to my friend's complaints and got an immediate picture of what was going on in her body. I drew my impressions and then focused on the area of the drawing that needed energetic attention. Using my pendulum and the map I created of my friend's distress, I was able to adjust the energy fields of her body and help her clear the sore throat.

This was the beginning of the basic procedure I now use. It doesn't matter whether the client is two feet away or two thousand miles away. I produce anywhere from three to ten draw-ings during an hour-long session. I treat each session as if I were physically with the client. The client schedules an appointment and I take a short history. Usually by the time I begin the interview, I've already received enough psychic information to begin. This technique is a powerful one. I do not recommend attempting long-distance healing without the help of a mentor. The telephone is a major conductor of energy, and one needs to learn how to deflect unwanted energy. If you feel absolutely compelled to do this, please be sure to draw your impressions. Somehow they seem to absorb unwanted energy, and they may act as a buffer. I usually destroy the drawings because they collect unwanted energy.

At times, long-distance healing and the drawings associated with the healings give additional information about physical and mental states. I was treating a woman with macular degeneration and discovered an area of distress in her foot. When I asked her if she had any problems in her feet she was taken aback by the information that I had received through the sketches.

The drawings can become an important diagnostic tool; the X's indicate the areas that need to be cleared. Once these areas are cleared, I infuse the cleared areas with energy. I've even used these sketches when MRIs did not provide the needed information. The areas of disturbance become very apparent in the drawings. Although I normally destroy the drawings of the sketches that I do, I have decided to include several sketches of a patient who was recovering from a brain tumor.

This patient was receiving treatment at Sloan Kettering hospital, which is approximately 3,000 miles away from where I conducted the healings. After sketch number one, the client was more energetic and relaxed. His wife verified this, as she was a witness to the healing.

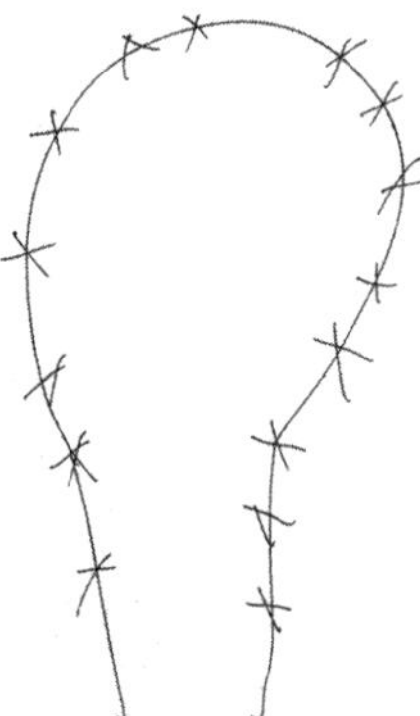

Sketch 1 (Simulation)

The second sketch was a very interesting one for me. As you can see, the page is filled with numerous X's. My sense about this drawing is that more subtle material would be dealt with and that the first sketch helped to clear the field. I sensed that toxins were being released in the second sketch. As with most digestive complaints, I was belching during the entire time I was working on him. He had been on steroids and a morphine drip, two very toxic drugs. At the end of the second sketch, I was more comfortable and, in fact, so was the client.

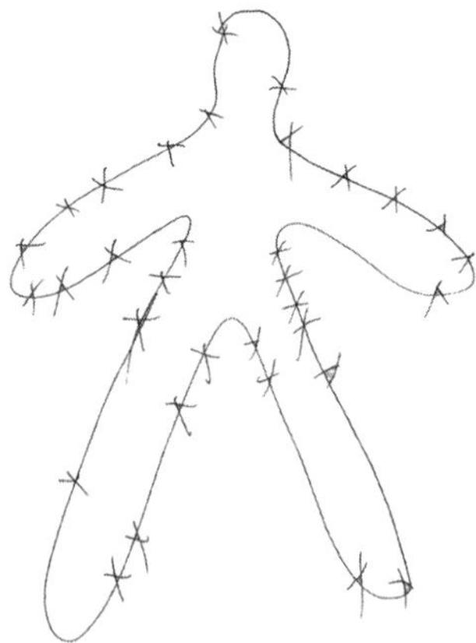

Sketch 2 (Simulation)

Another remarkable aspect of this particular healing is the fact that this client's speech returned to a normal cadence. Initially, the speech was very slow and flat. At the end of our conversation, it was apparent that his speech was quicker and more vibrant. The client was in a very weakened condition, and because of his fatigue level we broke phone contact after I got my initial impression.

These drawings were done the day after the patient had received his radiation treatment; he had been very fatigued and had vomited several times. My attempts with these drawings were just to re-energize the body. Once again, the wife observed that he experienced a positive change; his skin tone was more normal after the healings.

The Pendulum

I will only briefly discuss the use of the pendulum. It is a difficult technique in which the novice frequently gets incorrect information. It is truly a lovely tool that can help with pain, obtain details about food sensitivities, gain information about appropriate homeopathic and pharmaceutical treatments, help run energy through the body, and assist in conducting long-distance healing. There is a tremendous mystique about the pendulum. There are hand-carved wooden pendulums, crystals, and various pendants that are said to have special powers. In my trainings I try to demystify the use of the pendulum by suggesting that my students use a wet tea bag as a pendulum, as noted in Chapter 1. The students are usually surprised by the results they achieve with a modest tea bag. The evenness of the swing is the key to an efficient pendulum. And tea bags do just fine. Again, I don't feel it would be responsible of me to go into great detail about the pendulum. It requires time, patience, and diligence to become efficient with this precious tool, and it is not something that can be taught through a training manual.

I will note that in addition to healing work, there are other ways in which I use the pendulum. There was a particular instance I can recall when I was in the desert. All the sage and tumbleweed were looking alike, and I was having a difficult time recognizing the landmarks that would assist me in finding my way. I used my pendulum to determine the correct direction for exiting the area. Dowsing for a friend's lost contact lens was another useful application for the pendulum.

Healing Interaction

In your interaction with clients you will find that your intuition will probably be heightened. You may get flashes about certain behaviors or repetitive actions or reactions. Receiving the information intuitively is only a small part of your process. How valid is the information you have received? Is any of this information a projection of your own needs or desires? Let's assume that the information you have received is clear and accurate. What is the best way to communicate this information? Is this information meant to be communicated or is it information that is best kept to yourself?

Recently, I was having a conversation with a client who professed to be madly in love. We had just begun treatment and so it was necessary to ask a few questions to gain additional insight. I asked the client how long he had known his lover. He replied that even though he had only known her for two weeks he was madly in love and wanted to marry her. His eyes glistened as he told me that he had never felt anything like this before. As he said this I could sense the severe emotional disturbance in his beloved along with a diagnosis. I knew that if I had given this information to this bedazzled male at the time I would not only alienate him but he would never hear me. That being the case, I tucked this information away and discussed these distressing characteristics after the relationship was over.

When I am offering information to a client, I frequently try to do this in the form of an open-ended question. For instance, if I have received information that a husband is very controlling in a relationship I might ask, "How do you feel about equality in relationships?" The open-ended nature of this question helps the client come to independent conclusions and is a less threatening way to approach the situation. Let's look at the obvious question. How do you feel about controlling husbands? This could immediately put your client on the defensive and/or in denial and thus end the discussion.

The well-crafted open-ended question beautifully skirts the issue. How does one craft an open-ended question that will disarm the client and also elicit the needed information? Sometimes asking for an opinion will initiate important conversation. Another interesting way to broach a topic is to ask for quantification of the situation. For instance, "How severe is your emotional pain regarding your son?" The question is gently leading and also makes an assumption about the pain experienced in connection with a relationship or an incident or whatever. The client is less likely to deny a disturbance if a question is framed in this manner.

After you have gathered the information you require, how are you going to maintain the same gentleness as you analyze the data? If information is offered with an attitude of mutual respect it is much more likely to be received. You can ask your client if this information seems to fit. I find it useful to preface certain statements with "In my opinion, it seems to me…" or "Have you considered the possibility…" It makes you less of an expert and makes the relationship more of a partnership. The partnership allows for greater equality in the relationship and serves as a reminder for you that the work and healing energy will come through you. You are not the work.

Protection

There are numerous ways to deflect unwanted energy. Due to the fact that it is very easy to communicate an energy through the gaze, it is important for the practitioner to know how to address certain forms of eye contact. During a casual conversation, eye contact is intermittently maintained. In a therapeutic session, eye contact can be used to transmit an energy. This situation may begin to feel uncomfortable if the client is very compromised either physically or mentally.

My first experience of feeling uncomfortable occurred when I was treating a group of adolescent schizophrenics. I was teaching yoga at a mental hospital and began to feel very agitated. Fortunately, I was able to pinpoint the source of my agitation. The gaze of my adolescent students was penetrating, and unknowingly they were communicating a very disturbing energy. It is similar to the interaction you might have with an individual who has been using recreational drugs or has had too much to drink. There is a jaggedness and a jarring that I experience. I personally remove myself from these situations as quickly as I can. In the case of the adolescent students, my advice would be to avoid all eye contact.

It is too large of an energy to contend with. These are extreme examples of eye contact transmitting an unwanted energy.

In a therapeutic setting, if you find that you are experiencing an unwanted energy you can alter that interaction by merely looking to the left side, the right side, or the top of the head. The choice of looking to the left or right side will depend on how you are seated with your client. This technique allows you to be present with your client and yet you are not putting yourself in jeopardy by receiving unwanted energy.

Unwanted energy that is being communicated in ways other than the eyes can be deflected in several ways. One of the most basic ways to deflect unwanted energy is to wear white clothing. I find that wearing a long white shirt protects my chakras. I feel as if the energy is being deflected. If I am having a conversation with the client and suspect that an unwanted energy is being emitted I try to protect my heart and throat chakra. Frequently, I will support my elbow on a desk or the arm of a chair and cross my forearms against my chest. I rest my hand on my chin. The diagonal direction of my forearm conveniently protects the heart and throat chakra.

Another, but more obvious, way to block and deflect unwanted energy is to cross the forearms against the chest; this allows a counteracting energy to be released. If you are seated across from a client who is emitting an unwanted energy, feel free to position your chair so that you are not directly facing your client. If you place your chair so that you are slightly to the right or left of your client, the energy may become less intense. It is frequently helpful to actually move your chair so that you create a greater distance between you and your client.

If your client is lying down you may experience a release of energy from the pelvic area. If this is your experience, particularly with energy balancing, move to one side. You are most vulnerable when standing at the client's feet facing the head. Allow the energy to release and continue to stand to one side. If you have experienced unwanted energy, you may have a heavy feeling on your skin. It can cause fatigue, agitation, and restlessness.

If you feel you are experiencing unwanted energy there are several ways to reduce your uneasiness. Taking a salt water bath helps to reduce symptoms. Generally a cup of table salt or sea salt added to your bath water will relieve you of the negative energy. Make sure that you submerge your hair. For some reason, hair may hold an energy. In order to cleanse yourself, be sure to thoroughly wet your hair. If you are exposed to chemical toxicity such as pollution, an ounce of Clorox added to your bath water will cleanse your skin.

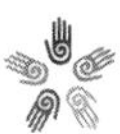

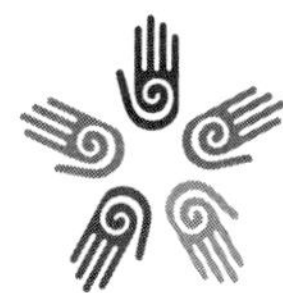

Chapter 9

Uncommon Solutions to Common Complaints

Stretches

Yoga Stretches

There are many postures and stretches that can help you correct body stresses and the disturbances that result from these stresses.

The Head, Neck, and Shoulders

One of the most effective movements for the head and neck is a very slow neck roll.

Sit in a chair and relax your body. Lower your head and continue to relax. Using the slowest possible movement, turn your head in a clockwise direction. This full rotation should take approximately sixty seconds. When you have completed your clockwise rotation, slowly begin a counterclockwise movement. This should also take sixty seconds. You will begin to feel as if your head is moving on its own volition. This exercise may be useful for eyestrain, pains in the neck, and headache; the slow movement can also have a relaxing effect. If at any time you begin to experience pain, reduce the magnitude of your rotation. The slow movement will protect you from injury or exacerbating any known injuries.

Another simple exercise for the head and neck involves moving the head and shoulders.

Sit in an upright position. Start on the right side. Drop your head to the right as you lift your shoulder. It is a shrugging motion. Return your head to a neutral position and drop your head to the left as you lift your left shoulder. Continue to alternate your movements. Develop a rhythm so that it feels like the ticking of a clock. This gently massages the neck and helps to increase mobility.

The yoga mudra may help to release stress in the head and neck.

Place your hands on your thighs. This may be done standing or in a kneeling position. Very slowly allow your hands to lift from your thighs. Let them slowly float in a circle until you are clasping your hands behind you. If you are very flexible, you may straighten your arms. The emphasis, however, will be on moving the shoulder blades towards each other. This helps to open the chest and will frequently give you the releases you are looking for in the neck. This exercise is done very slowly and with an attitude of reverence. When the hands are released, you will feel a lightness and the hands will feel as if they are moving on their own volition. This slow motion helps to fool the body so sometimes you may experience unexpected releases. One of my students had chronic neck problems and this exercise helped to shift her to another plateau of mobility.

Another potent stretch for the neck and shoulders also opens up the chest.

Stand with your feet about six inches apart. Gaze at the floor about four to six feet from your body. Have a neutral expression on your face. Raise your right arm until it is parallel with the floor. Have your palm facing the floor. Keeping your alignment, extend your energy into your middle finger. Turn your palm up and reach for the ceiling. Try to lift your rib cage as you reach for the ceiling. Ideally, your arm should be upright and close to your ear. Stay active in the pose by continuing to stretch toward the ceiling. To come out of the pose, lower your entire arm and continue to extend energy through your middle finger. Turn the palm downward and lower your arm to your side. Wait for fifteen to thirty seconds before you repeat on the other side. This is a very simple stretch and at the same time an exceedingly engaging one. Your chest is enlivened, and your arms are strengthened. It helps with overall alignment and helps to release tension in the neck. I recommend that you pause for thirty to sixty seconds before you go on to another stretch. I call this time one of recalibration. The energy freely moves through your body and nourishes the areas of deficit.

It is important to move the energy through the neck, arms, and spine.

Stand facing the wall. Place your hands on the wall so that your fingertips are parallel to the tops of your shoulders. Take a step backward and flatten your back. Form a ninety-degree angle with your back and your legs. With your feet firmly planted try to lift the buttocks, maintaining a flat back. Apply a light pressure to the wall and be sure to maintain contact with the wall. Keep the fingers equidistant and have the middle finger pointing upright. This hand gesture is very useful in preventing arthritis. As you can imagine, you are engaging the spine, shoulders, and neck. The active legs stretch the hamstrings, and the altitude of the hand will increase flexibility.

The Abdomen

A useful exercise for massaging the abdomen and intestines can be performed seated in a chair or kneeling on the floor.

Clasp your elbows and bend forward. You will feel a slight pressure on the abdomen or the intestines. This posture may help to stimulate a bowel movement. It is excellent for menstrual cramps, relieving gas, and enlivening the intestines. It is also useful with individuals who have taken medication that has a constipating effect. Many years ago, I worked in a methadone clinic. Methadone is a synthetic opiate and is very constipating. This technique proved to be successful in the treatment of this medically induced distress.

Hand Exercises

The flower is a useful exercise for the treatment of arthritis in the hand.

> The flower consists of gently opening and closing each hand. As you slowly close your hand, make sure that your thumb is tucked into your palm. Slowly open and close as frequently as you'd like.

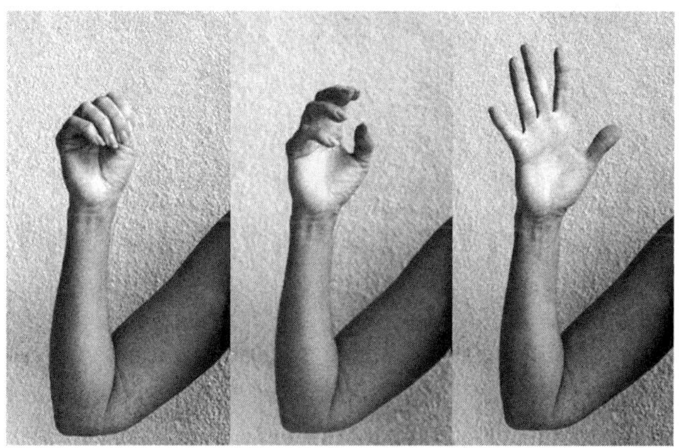

Pelvis, Back, Abdomen, and Knees

One of my favorite subtle stretches addresses the pelvis, back, abdomen, and knees, and may help with alignment.

> Lie on your back with your hands at your sides. Begin by paying attention to your right foot. Using the outside of your right foot, slowly drag it on the floor until you have reached the area where you think your knee is. Flatten your foot and place your foot on the floor. Hold this position for the count of three and then lower your foot once again using the outside of your foot. Pause for a moment and then repeat on the left side. Pause for a moment and repeat using both feet. You will look like a tadpole.

I have used this very gentle exercise with individuals who had badly arthritic knees. It releases tightness in the knees and increases flexibility. There are situations in which neck pain is decreased with this attention to the lower body.

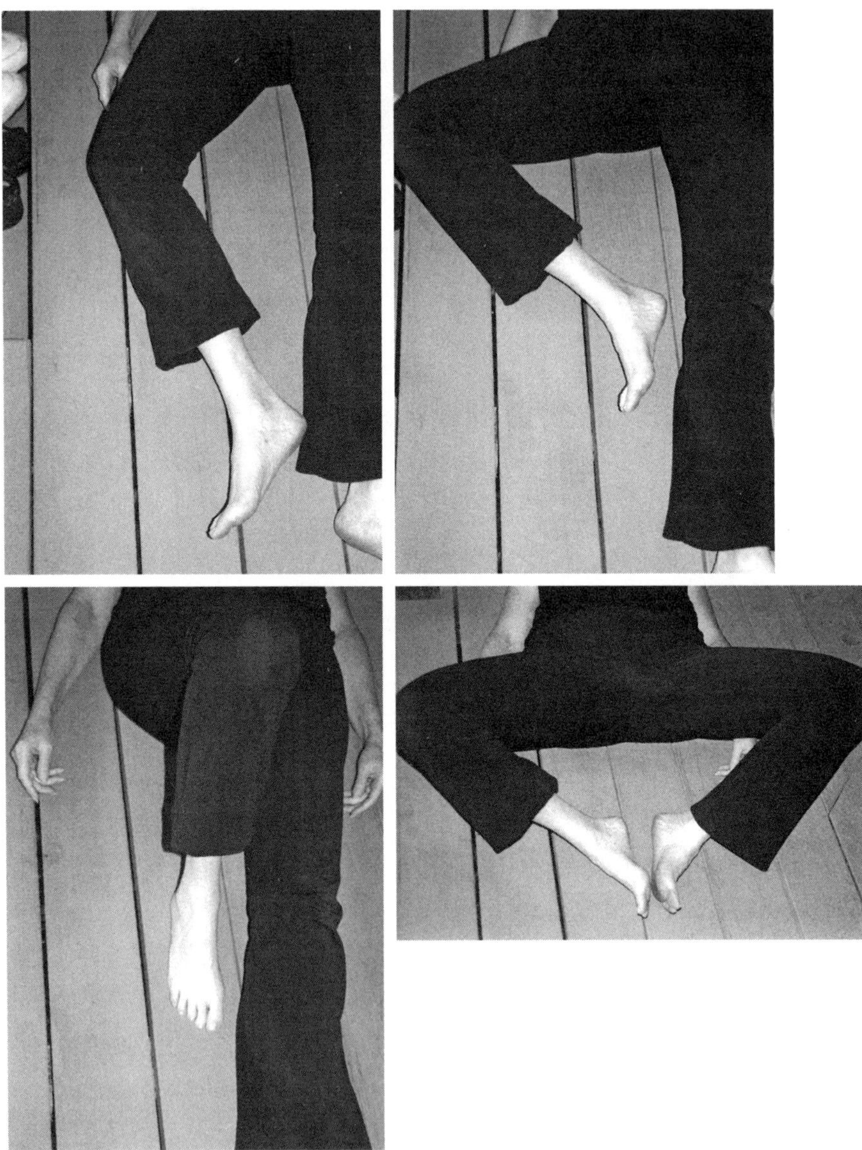

The Feet

Another simple but subtle exercise has to do with bringing energy to the feet.

As you walk very slowly and purposefully, lift your heels and spread your toes. The more the heels lift to the ceiling, the more flexible the toes become. This exercise helps with balance and correcting stiffness in the feet. This slow movement also has a calming effect. The feet are usually not noticed until they become painful. This slow meditation walk can be used prophylactically to encourage balance and move energy to the feet. If you choose to have a soft focus, gaze four to six feet in front of you, and you will have the additional effect of relaxing the face.

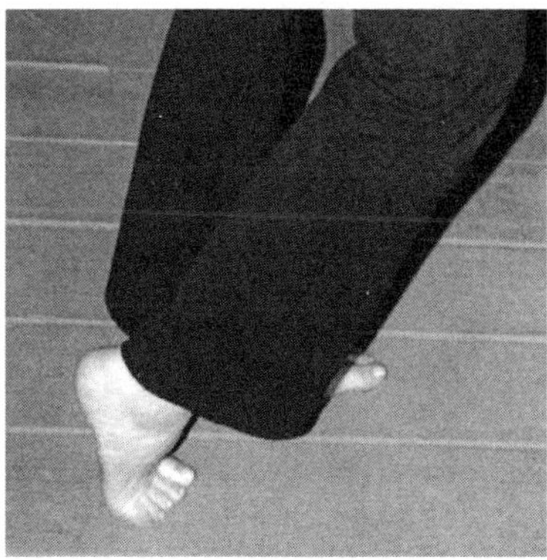

An interesting way to infuse energy into the foot is to clasp the feet.

Place the palm of your hand against the ball of your foot. Interlace your fingers between your toes. Place your little finger in between your little toe and your fourth toe. Keep entwining your fingers until you have interlaced all of your fingers. Gently and slowly move your toes forward and backward. Make sure that you use the hand opposite the foot that you are massaging. Repeat on the other side. This technique enlivens the entire foot. I have recommended this exercise to individuals who were recovering from foot and ankle surgeries. Generally, this is something not to be done immediately after surgery but rather to alleviate some of the stiffness that frequently occurs after surgery. It is also useful for improving balance. After surgery, the non-involved foot usually is overworked and this ultimately can affect balance. If you see that this is the case, do the exercise on the over-worked side. Hopefully, this will help with the correction.

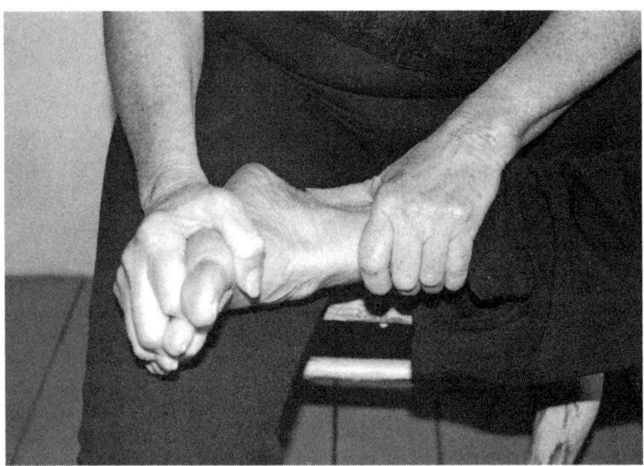

Centering

There are several techniques that I would recommend for centering. Some involve more of a mental process than a physical one.

Candle Gazing

Sit in front of the flame of a household candle. Study the flame in great detail. Observe how it moves. Observe how it changes in color. Observe the glow surrounding the flame. Continue to observe the flame for approximately thirty seconds. Close your eyes and observe the afterimage. You will probably see a negative image. With your eyes closed, continue to observe the afterimage. When the afterimage has faded, open your eyes and once again observe the nuances of the flame. Repeat this process until your mind quiets. One of the advantages of a technique such as this is that you have a point of focus. It is much easier to quiet the mind when attention can be paid directly to an object.

Sense Withdrawal

This technique is based on the yoga principle of sense withdrawal.

Sit at a table or any seated position in which you can comfortably put your elbows on a table. Place your thumbs in your ears, your index and middle finger on your eyelids, and your forth finger just below your nostrils. The placement of the fourth finger is a symbolic closing off of your sense of smell. Once you have comfortably positioned your hands and your elbows, begin to hum. The humming sound will vibrate through your ears and begin to change your concentration. With the sound vibrating through your head, it is difficult to think disturbing thoughts or thoughts that involve cognitive thinking. For instance, shopping lists, to-do lists, and the checkbook are items that cannot physically be addressed. The sound bypasses the cognitive process. It is a lovely technique for thought stopping.

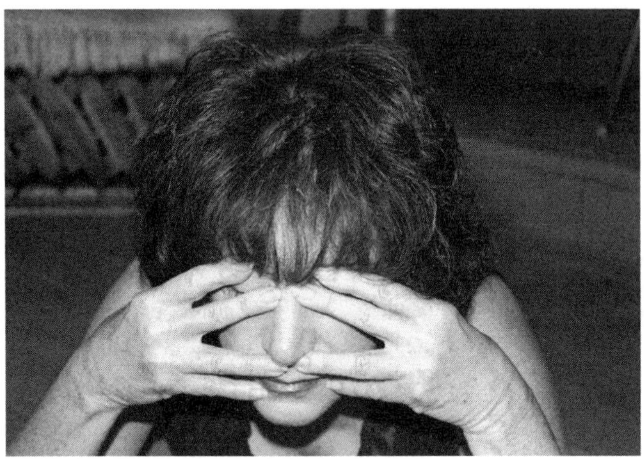

Sense Withdrawal

The Golden Cross

This exercise quiets both the mind and the body.

Stand with your feet close together unless you feel that you need to separate your feet for balance. Raise your arms to the side so that they are parallel to the floor. Move energy through your middle fingers. Gaze softly at the floor. Hold the position until you feel yourself quiet or your arms are exhausted. If you return your arms to your sides because they are tired, lift them as soon as they are rested and repeat the exercise until you feel centered.

Home Remedies

Sinus Congestion

Sinus congestion can be a very annoying condition. In addition to experiencing stuffiness in the head, it can also contribute to fatigue, headaches, irritability, and brain fog. Sinus conditions can affect the teeth and cause painful gums; it also can lead to congestion in the ears and hearing loss. This condition can be a very elusive one as there are many causes of sinus congestion. Environmental stressors may include mold, pollen, pollution, and dust. Ingested stressors may include food, alcohol, and even vitamins and herbal supplements. Regardless of the cause, it is essential to clear the nasal passages.

One way to clear the nasal passages is based on an ancient yoga kriya.

> Add one-half teaspoon of salt to an eight-ounce glass of lukewarm water. Dissolve the salt as best you can. With your head over a basin, pour the lightly salted water into your hand. Bring your hand to your nostril and try to inhale the lightly salted water one side at a time. Obviously, this is a rather messy process and you will probably appreciate your basin. Try to repeat this three to four times daily for acute cases. This should afford you immediate relief.

Acupuncture points can also be helpful in clearing symptoms. The areas on the eyebrows are very useful points to begin with. One point that can be very telling is the point at the inner end of the eyebrow. This is one point that can be particularly painful if the sinuses are inflamed. Maintain a moderate pressure on these points. The difference between what we will be doing and traditional acupressure is the fact that our intention will be to use healing energy to open these resistant areas. The three main points on the eyebrows are on the innermost part of the eyebrow, the indentation about two-thirds near the end of the eyebrow and the end of the eyebrow. These points are particularly useful if your client is complaining of sinus headache. The points by the sides of the nostrils are very important for reducing nasal congestion. Initially, these points may be very tender, so please proceed with a light touch. The uppermost part of the cheek has another very significant point.

Another technique for clearing the sinuses has to do with manual manipulation of the fingers.

On either side of each finger you will find a thickening. When a thickening feels uneven from side to side, put pressure on the thicker side. You have probably found a sinus point on your finger that relates to the sinus points on your face. You can actually open the points on the face by working the fingers. It's a very impressive technique that you can share with your clients. It is one of the few techniques that can be done by the client with the same results that would be achieved with a practitioner.

Certain foods can also contribute to sinus congestion.

There is a general consensus that dairy products, milled flours, and alcohol can be culprits in creating additional mucous. I would recommend that these items be eliminated until conditions clear.

Digestive Complaints

Digestive complaints usually fall into one of two categories: acute or chronic. Digestive complaints that are acute usually require immediate attention. For instance, occasional constipation can be treated herbally. For immediate relief, one or two capsules of aloe vera usually get the system moving within twelve hours. It is a very potent herb when taken in capsule form. If a persistent condition exists, the dosage will need to be regulated. Frequently, one capsule every other day or half a capsule daily will keep the system moving. Because of its healing properties, in many cases it can be ultimately used on an as-needed basis.

Prune juice is a remedy that is quite standard. However, the potency can be boosted by heating and drinking it slowly. Because the properties in prune juice are more remedial than healing, I would suggest using aloe vera capsules for chronic conditions with the hope that the healing benefits of aloe vera would reduce the chronic nature of the constipation.

If the actual flora of the colon needs to be boosted, a high grade of acidophilus is frequently useful. Most health food stores have a refrigerated section of high-potency acidophilus. If you have taken antibiotics, it is likely that the flora in your system has been disturbed. I highly recommend that you immediately begin taking acidophilus to correct this condition.

Occasional diarrhea can be treated in several ways. If the case of diarrhea is mild, it is frequently a good idea to just let it run its course. If in twenty-four hours you have not recovered or if the frequency or consistency of the stool is troublesome, the simplest approach is an over-the-counter preparation.

For cases of long-standing or intermittent diarrhea, other interventions must be considered. The case of chronic diarrhea must be investigated, and dehydration must be avoided, particularly when young children and advanced seniors are involved. Chronic diarrhea can have many causes. Nearly twenty-five years ago, I was introduced to a very forward-thinking physician who looked at environmental stressors and allergens as factors contributing to gastrointestinal complaints. When we think of allergic reactions, we most frequently think about runny noses. Some individuals react to those same allergens with a gastrointestinal complaint. If this is the case, allergy testing is sometimes useful, and certainly eliminating those identified stressors will be helpful.

Gastrointestinal complaints resulting from parasites should be attended to in yet another way. If symptoms are severe, lab work is certainly helpful in identifying the parasite. I personally have had many episodes of parasite infestation. My earliest recollection was related to my travels to Costa Rica. I also was struck in London. One does not have to be in a Third World country to experience parasites. You can get parasites in a fast food restaurant or a five-star restaurant. They are present and prevalent everywhere.

If you suspect that you have parasites, grapefruit seed extract tablets may be helpful. Grapefruit seed extract comes in several forms; tablets are most efficient for dealing with intestinal parasites. Parasites cannot only cause diarrhea but also mucous in the stools, blood in the stools, bloating, constipation, and nausea. I recommend taking immediate action if you suspect parasites. If your symptoms subside and you are not treated, the parasites can become dormant but still present. Parasites are usually most active during the full moon. If you regularly experience digestive distress during the full moon you may become suspicious. Try heavy doses of grapefruit seed extract, and if you become uncomfortable, you may be passing the critters.

Intense bloating may accompany parasite infestation. If this is the case, try ginger compresses for the abdomen. This is also useful for cramping. Add four tablespoons of ground or fresh ginger to two quarts of boiling water. Let steep for five minutes. Dip a washcloth into the water and wring out. Place on abdomen and repeat for ten minutes. This may also help to relieve gas and the associated gas pains. Another useful intervention for gas and nausea is vinegar water. To an eight-ounce glass of warm water add one teaspoon of apple cider vinegar and sip slowly and repeat in one half-hour if symptoms persist.

Another very simple solution for gastric distress is the use of caraway seeds and Umeboshi plum pits. In both cases, the client sucks on the seeds and the pits. The caraway seeds can be chewed after they lose their initial potency, and the Umeboshi plum pits can be sucked on indefinitely. The saliva produced by sucking on the pits produce a very alkaline environment and helps to ease the gastric distress.

Herbs and Such

Siberian Ginseng has therapeutic properties that are truly unique. The anti-inflammatory character of Siberian Ginseng can be used for joints and other areas of inflammation due to injury and infection. If used therapeutically, it has properties that are similar to some steroids and in some cases can be used in their place. Therefore, it is a valuable aid in assisting individuals to wean from steroids. The side effects of steroids can be very challenging, including weakened bones, a moon-like face, moodiness, and a compromised immune system. Therefore, I strongly urge the introduction of Siberian Ginseng with the hope that steroid use can be diminished.

Siberian Ginseng has few side effects. If you have high blood pressure or any irregular heart conditions, certainly consult a physician before using Siberian Ginseng. It is definitely a stimulant and certain precautions should be taken. Siberian Ginseng comes in different strengths, and I normally recommend taking two to eight capsules daily. I think that it is necessary to start with a lesser amount initially and slowly build your levels. Because it is a stimulant, it can affect your heartbeat.

Siberian Ginseng has the ability to boost the immune system. If taken regularly for a period of four to six weeks, you may find that certain allergic reactions are diminished. This is an energizing herb and will probably make you feel energetic. It is also purported to have particular value in boosting a masculine energy. I am not specifically recommending Siberian Ginseng as an aphrodisiac, but it does have a masculine flavor to it.

Dong Quai is a feminine booster. It may aid in the production of estrogen. It is contraindicated, however, if a high estrogen is problematic. Many times fibroids are associated with elevated estrogen levels. If this is the case, Dong Quai would not be the herb of choice. Dong Quai can also increase energy. It can be used to combat menopausal symptoms and PMS. It helps to regulate estrogen and keep the mind clear and focused.

Valerian root is used as a sedative. It has many of the properties that Valium has. It can be used to ease a traumatic response or it can be used for a longer period of time to correct muscle spasm. It is frequently useful in relieving back pain. The tincture form is preferred by some and pill or tablet by others. This herb works on the central nervous system and helps to create an ease in the body. Therefore, it can be used in place of muscle relaxants.

Unfortunately, Valerian root has a very pungent, unpleasant odor, and if available the pill form seems to be less noxious. Valerian root is often found in combination with other sedative herbs such as Passion Flower and Chamomile.

There is some controversy as to whether Valerian root can contribute to a rapid heartbeat. There has also been discussion regarding the possibility that Valerian root is addictive. I personally do not believe it is addictive. However, if there is a predisposition to a heart irregularity, I generally do not recommend this herb.

Homeopathic Remedies

Homeopathic Cell Salts

There are many books for lay use on homeopathy. Many of them are quite useful, and yet I believe that the layperson needs to be cautious about using high-potency remedies and many remedies other than the cell salts. The cell salts are the most benign of the remedies and yet exceedingly effective. In low potencies, homeopathic cell salts are benign, and the only side effect that has ever been reported to me was sleepiness. My use of these remedies is not at all a classical approach. Over the years, I have developed a protocol that seems to work.

Due to the fact that I am not a physician, it is very important that I phrase my recommendations in a way that will not be construed as practicing medicine. This disclaimer pertains to any suggestions having to do with vitamins, herbs, and homeopathic remedies. The correct way to make a recommendation is to say, "It is thought, known, believed, etc. that so and so may be useful with your condition." With this in mind, I want to further state that I am not a homeopathic practitioner nor do I represent myself in that way. I do, however, refer to six homeopathic cell salts for use with common complaints.

The six cell salts that I use are:

Ferrum Phos

Kali Phos

Kali Mur

Nat Mur

Mag Phos

Nat Phos

Ferrum Phos

In my opinion, Ferrum Phos is the most important of these six cell salts. I often joke that if I were on a desert island, Ferrum Phos is the one homeopathic remedy that I would want to have. Ferrum Phos can be used prophylactically and to treat serious disorders. It promotes all types of healing; it can help reduce the symptoms of a common cold as well as to heal broken bones. If used as a paste, it can help to clear acne, reduce dermatitis, and reduce the itch from insect bites.

If I am exposed to a contagious condition, I take Ferrum Phos while I am treating my client. Ferrum Phos works on conditions that are both bacterial and viral in nature. I have recommended Ferrum Phos for stubborn ear infections that would not respond to antibiotics.

Recently, I recommended that one of my female clients take Ferrum Phos to prevent urinary tract infections. If Ferrum Phos is taken before sexual activity, UTI may not develop. Ferrum Phos can be used with any infectious condition, including sinus conditions (when green mucous is present), certain vaginal distresses, infected open wounds, and sore throats. It is an amazing remedy and very much underused. These remedies can be purchased at many health food stores, and each remedy is approximately $6. As you can imagine, no one makes any money on these over-the-counter remedies. Consequently, few if any advertising dollars are spent on educating the public about these little-known cell salts. These remedies are also available by mail through Santa Monica Pharmacy.

Kali Phos

The next cell salt that in itself is a gem is Kali Phos. This addresses deficiencies in the nervous system. I have recommended this for many conditions related to a compromised nervous system. It is useful in treating anxiety, depression, and insomnia. Some of the most stunning results of using Kali Phos have been with depression. I have recommended Kali Phos to bipolar patients who were resistant to pharmaceuticals. Sometimes this homeopathy can be used to boost the effects of pharmaceuticals. This notion will probably be very disturbing to practitioners who have been classically trained. However, I have found my unorthodox approach along with energetic healing to be very effective in many cases.

Kali Phos may help reduce night sweats associated with menopause. It is also known to be useful in treating PMS. When symptoms are severe, I recommend using 200x rather than a lower potency. Agitation resulting from exposure to environmental toxicity may also respond to Kali Phos. If you have been driving in heavy traffic or have experienced air pollution, Kali Phos may be useful in restoring balance to the body.

Kali Mur

Another very potent cell salt is Kali Mur. This is very specific and does not have the multiple uses that Kali Phos and Ferrum Phos do. This is specific for yellow or white mucous conditions. My former secretary had a very runny nose and was feeling just awful. Within minutes after she started taking Kali Mur the character of her distress changed. Her sinuses cleared and her face brightened. She was immediately relieved of her symptoms. The relief was short-lived, and in acute conditions the dose needs to be repeated every thirty minutes. With a cold or runny nose, Kali Mur is very helpful in reducing symptoms. In the case of chronic sinus congestion, I recommend using this remedy daily for a period of several months. Chronic conditions require a different approach for healing to take place.

Nat Mur

Nat Mur can be used to balance all water conditions. It can be used for dry mouth and dry skin. It can be used to counteract dry mouth that frequently accompanies anti-depressant use. One client decided to use Nat Mur when she experienced dry mouth and dry eyes during her desert travels. Her conditions used to be so severe and her frequent visits to her sister's desert house were always a challenge for her until she discovered the wonders of Nat Mur. Nat Mur is also used for allergic conditions in which there is a clear watery discharge from the nose.

Nat Mur is good for bloating and swollen ankles. It can act as a mild diuretic as it balances the water in the body. When I owned Casa Glorietta, I recommended it for mild constipation and dry skin. Although constipation and dry skin seem to have no relationship, both of these conditions are water conditions that require balance.

Mag Phos

Mag Phos is another interesting remedy. Mag Phos works on muscle spasm and sprains. This remedy may be very useful in controlling pain associated with spasm. Sometimes it is useful with headache or menstrual cramping. A unique characteristic of Mag Phos is that it can be taken in large quantities at bedtime. An individual can ingest one-eighth to one-fourth of a teaspoon, and hopefully it will alleviate morning stiffness in the back.

Nat Phos

Nat Phos is the last cell salt that I will discuss. Nat Phos is used specifically for acid indigestion, nausea, and a general stomach malaise.

Administration

Feel free to follow the instructions on the bottle. For adults, individuals may ingest four tabs four times daily. Children will take anywhere between one to two tabs four times daily. I mentioned that my use of cell salts is rather unorthodox and I violate the classical instructions. I believe that the most essential aspect of administration is to get the cell salts in the body. When clients need to wait one-half-hour after meals to avoid coffee, certain aromas, and peppermint, I find that there is not only resistance but in fact people just don't do it.

My instructions are to wait five minutes before or after you have had something in your mouth. Keep them on hand so that you have no excuse for not popping them. Try to avoid coffee right before or after you take them and don't take them right before or after you brush your teeth. One of my clients who was being treated by a classical practitioner inquired whether there were any smells of peppermint in my office. This again is a very classical approach. In acute cases, remedies can be taken every fifteen minutes for relief of symptoms.

As previously stated, my recommendation regarding potencies is cautious. The only high-potency remedies I use are Kali Phos and Ferrous Phos. Ferrous Phos can be used when antibiotics are not effective, and Kali Phos can be useful for stubborn cases of insomnia or depression.

Homeopathic cell salts can also be used in combination. The unorthodox way to combine homeopathic remedies is to ingest them all at once. The classical method requires that you wait one-half hour in between the remedies.

The following scenarios will help to give you a feel of how the cell salts can be used.

Scenario 1:

A young adult has a runny nose and a high fever. What remedies would you use? Before combining remedies, it is most important to determine the character of the discharge from the nose. Is the mucous clear, white, or green? Remember that your choice of remedy will depend on those findings. Regarding treatment of the fever, it is fairly safe to assume that Ferrum Phos would be a good choice.

Scenario 2:

An individual has a complaint of back pain and stiffness that is most pronounced in the A.M. You may begin with the usual dose of Mag Phos but also consider a mega dose at bed time that would include a one-eighth to one-fourth teaspoon of Mag Phos.

Scenario 3:

A twelve-month-old baby has an earache. What are you going to do? Very cautiously try one tab of Ferrum Phos every two to four hours. The potency should be 3x or 6x. If the child does not appear better in several hours, please check with your physician. In my unorthodox opinion, I believe that homeopathic remedies can boost pharmaceuticals, so if your physician prescribes an antibiotic, feel free to continue with the homeopathic remedy.

Scenario 4:

Your best friend is scheduled for surgery and she is a nervous wreck. Kali Phos is very useful for calming individuals. For an adult, I would begin with 30x, and if this is not effective try 200x. Follow the instructions for acute cases if in fact this appears to be acute, or use a maintenance dose if the symptoms are ongoing. Ferrum Phos is also very useful for healing. It may be used with pre-surgical conditions as it enriches and enlivens the cells before surgery. It is very useful after surgery as it promotes healing. It also is useful in preventing and reducing infections associated with post-surgical conditions.

Scenario 5:

It is allergy season and you are secreting a clear discharge. Nat Mur is the remedy of choice. I would also like to add dietary recommendations. Avoid dairy and wheat products. If possible try a fruit fast for a day or two. If the allergic reactions become chronic, you may experience sinusitis. If this is the case and the mucous turns yellow or white, try Kali Mur. If it turns green, add Ferrum Phos to the Kali Mur or Nat Mur.

There are several other remedies I would like to include in this discussion. Arnica is very useful for trauma and injury. It provides healing and may reduce black and blue marks. Nux vomicus is useful for many types of stomach upsets. It can be used for acid indigestion, constipation, belching, and a general feeling of fullness. Calm and Calm Forte are two combinations manufactured by Hyland. These are frequently useful for insomnia and nervous conditions. Nerve Tonic, also manufactured by Hyland, assists with nervous exhaustion and sleeplessness. This combination remedy will also give a gentle boost if energy is lagging due to exhaustion and overwork.

Rescue Remedy is in an entirely different category. It is a Bach flower combination and can be used with many types of trauma. It can be used for pre- and post-surgical conditions as well as stresses associated with relationships including professional and personal relationships. It is a liquid and can be ingested, or you may add it to water or even rub it on your wrist. In the case of post-surgical patients, it is sometimes necessary to use this remedy only on the wrist. I generously applied it to my wrists during a very trying, tedious court hearing. It has a calming effect and allows you to function as if there were less trauma.

These potent remedies are exceedingly useful, and in the many years that I have been using them, I still marvel at the rapid changes that occur with their use.

Partner Healing

I would like to share simple, safe ways to communicate energy to a partner who has been physically compromised due to illness, injury, surgery, or advanced aging.

The psychological adjustments that accompany a physical compromise can be very challenging to integrate into one's psyche. The body that once was is not the one that has experienced the physical assault. For instance, I have worked with many recovering cancer patients who have had breast surgeries. The surgeries have ranged from lumpectomies to double mastectomies, and the manner in which the patients deal with their procedures vary greatly.

One woman who had a double mastectomy proudly and defensively announced that she had no breasts. She felt like a boy and began to swagger in a masculine way. When we carefully examined her incised areas we were actually able to see some breast tissue. We neutrally viewed the remaining breast tissue and after a few sessions of soul searching, the masculine swagger diminished.

Another woman who had a double mastectomy felt like a butterfly after her surgery. She could spread her wings and had no fear about further breast cancers. She enjoyed her freedom and had no obvious issues with her femininity or identity.

For couples who are experiencing trauma from illness, injury, or other conditions, some very straightforward, safe, and simple techniques may be useful. I want to emphasize that in a relationship, the trauma of the physically compromised individual is also experienced by the unaffected partner. For instance, after heart surgery (it seems that more men than women have heart surgery) the female partner can feel very separate from her partner. The fears associated with a physical exchange after a surgery of this nature is present for both parties. This, however, is the precise time when partners need each other and a physical closeness.

A safe technique that encourages physical closeness involves lying back-to-back. The spine acts as a conduit, and the energy flows through the spine. When the spines connect in this manner, the energy intermingles.

If partners are strong enough, the more desirable position is to be seated in a cross-legged position. The more complete the connection, the more the energy will be able to intermingle. This technique requires that you remain still for several minutes. Most couples experience a peaceful, supportive energy during this exercise.

Another technique calls for partners to sit in chairs. Each partner places the right hand on the middle of the partner's sternum. This technique stimulates the heart chakra, which is located at the sternum. Be still for a few minutes as the energy gathers. A more tactile technique involves spooning. Both partners lie in a fetal-like position. One partner wraps around the other partner. The partner whose back is exposed becomes active in this technique. The activity requires stimulating the chakras through touch. Once again, place the hand on the heart chakra and hold for several minutes. Move to the top of the head and hold. Move to the solar plexus and hold. Move to the genitals and hold. Allow the energy to gather and change position and roles.

Analyzing and Treating Depression and Anxiety

Depression and anxiety are most frequently treated without taking into account physical imbalances. It has been my experience that most depression is accompanied by physical disturbances in the skull. Most situations of panic anxiety can be traced to an imbalance in the chest cavity. This can be associated with imbalances in the rib cage, the sternum, or in some cases the clavicle. Symmetry once again plays a large part in allowing the energy to move freely through the body.

I have treated many stubborn cases of depression that were resistant to medication. By placing my hands on either side of the skull, I am usually able to trace the imbalance contributing to the depression.

One client describes her sense of depressive assault as if there were a chard of glass piercing her skull. The pressure of the imbalances in her skull causes her to feel as if she is out of control. When she no longer experiences that pressure, life is manageable for her. We have been working together for six months and her episodes of depression are nominal. The more balance she experiences in her physical body, the more balance she experiences in her mood.

I personally have had the experience of how the balance in the cranium can affect mood. Several years ago, I was involved in an automobile accident. I was a passenger in the first car of a three-car, rear-end collision. I had a slight concussion, which immediately affected my mood. Within a few days of the accident, I experienced an unusual irritability. I also experienced symptoms of depression and lethargy. The concussion caused an instability in my cranial bones, and it took over a year to be symptom-free. It was quite an eye-opener for me. Energetic healing has consistently been useful in dealing with depression, and before my episode I had thought that the energy acted to transform cells in ways that naturally simulated the effects of anti-depressants. I still believe that this is the case, but now I have discovered that stability in the cranium reduces symptoms of depression. My clients verify this by reporting symptoms coinciding with feelings of imbalance and discomfort.

Anxiety also seems to have a physical component. The daughter of a physician had tried many pharmaceuticals and psychotherapy to relieve her symptoms of anxiety. By the time that we connected she had exhausted all known medical interventions to control her symptoms. At our first meeting, we chatted and she described some of her panic anxiety episodes. It was difficult for her to have a social life. She was sometimes overcome with anxiety in restaurants, theaters, and parties. At times she would feel compelled to leave the event because she couldn't catch her breath. As we were talking, I could see the imbalances in her chest. I asked her if she would allow me to show her the imbalances. I touched her on either side of her sternum and she was able to feel the origin of her difficulty. Frequently, it is easier to work on a corresponding area than directly on the area of distress. If I had dropped a plum line from back to front I would have been directly on the area of distress. The woman's symptoms were completely manageable after three sessions, and after a few months she was stable and totally symptom-free. Her anxiety was directly related to the imbalance in her chest. We remained in contact for many months, and her episodes of panic anxiety were eradicated.

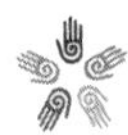

Chapter 10

UCLA:
The Classroom Experiences

As I mentioned in Section I, I had the pleasure of lecturing at UCLA's School of Medicine. I can remember how anxious I was first pulling into the underground parking lot of the UCLA medical center. I wanted this class to work, and I didn't know how I would be received. Would these first-year medical students even have an interest in what I had to say? Susan Stangl, M.D., who introduced me to the students, assured me that there was a strong interest in the work.

After introductions and an explanation of hands-on-healing, I instructed the students in a technique that brings energy to the hands (described in Chapter 8: Healing for Beginners). The students were attentive and almost all of them experienced a sensation in their hands. Any remaining skepticism was dissipated by this experience. The students had many questions about the application of energy to medical complaints. Their curiosity was piqued, and I felt that the lecture was a success.

As a result of the lecture/demonstration, I proposed an educational series. Dr. Stangl was happy to have me join in the selective program. Although I received no financial compensation for my services, the students were able to get credit for taking the class.

I structured the classes to include lecture, experiential exercises, and my clients' discussions about their personal experiences with healing energy. The inclusion of these guest speakers made a huge impression on the students; they were able to ask questions and gain valuable insight.

Gail's Family Healer

I've been Gail's family healer for many years. Gail had a number of presenting complaints. She had had a bout with mononucleosis, and as a result her immune system was depressed. She had chronic neck and back pain. She was easily fatigued and had gastrointestinal distresses. Gail was also stressed by her working conditions and actually arranged for me to do a stress-reduction workshop for the faculty at the high school where she was a teacher.

Gail and I met regularly for six months. Gail's reaction to the work was not typical. She usually experienced a delayed reaction to the treatment, and it was only after two or three days that she began to get relief from her symptoms. Gail's immune system seemed to perk up. She experienced less fatigue and stress. Her pains diminished, and she began to have a much healthier aura surrounding her.

I soon found myself working on Gail's friends and family. Bob, Gail's long-time friend, had problems with his knees as a result of football injuries. He had developed a bone spur and had tried many different forms of therapy in an attempt to correct his difficulties. Within a few sessions he was pain-free and returned to his treating physician. His physician took X-rays and found that there was no longer evidence of the bone spur.

On another occasion, Bob had stepped on a piece of glass and it became embedded in his foot. He tried soaking the foot and used various poultices. Nothing seemed to work. I was not very hopeful about anything that I could do for him; however, I treated him and his pain totally diminished. He thinks that the glass actually changed its composition and dispersed.

Gail's presentation was very well received. She answered many questions and advised the students to keep an open mind about healers. We continued the class discussion; the students brought up many concerns, some of which were of a personal nature. One student was interested in ways in which he could take care of himself while a medical student. He was concerned about picking up negative energy from the hospital and his patients.

Multiple Complaints Associated with Cancer

I met Joyce at the UCLA coffee shop before we went to class. She was beaming. Just prior to our meeting, she had been examined by her oncologist. Her physician was very pleased with her progress. We were both relieved to hear that her chest and arm pains were muscular and not related to a cancerous condition.

We entered the classroom and I began my lecture with an overview of how healers can work directly side-by-side with physicians effectively.

Joyce began her story of medical intervention. Her multiple surgeries ended in a radical mastectomy on the left side. After surgery, she experienced intense pain in the left quadrant, and the pain traveled to her fingertips. My first session with her addressed this situation. The pain subsided in several days, and with multiple treatments it was resolved.

Joyce had many fine surgeons who probably saved her life. My part in her recovery had to do with easing her pain and strengthening her immune system. She also experienced an emotional shift through our work. She couldn't put her finger on it, but she felt much better. Her co-workers remarked that she was looking better and younger.

During our last session, I was drawn to her left side. There was a slight elevation in the left side and as I began to infuse that side of her body; she began to feel a tingling sensation in her left foot and ankle. Her left ankle and leg were swollen. She had never mentioned this to me, and yet the energy found its way to where it was needed. The students were intrigued with this process; however, I was unable to give them any technical answers to their questions.

Self-Care for the Medical Student

At another session we discussed self-care and stress reduction. We talked about student stresses and how disturbing stress can be to the mind-body experience. Acknowledging that individuals have certain weaknesses, we discussed how these weaknesses act as magnets and collect stress during difficult periods. We identified areas of stress among the students. My intent was to increase awareness and assure students that stress was a significant part of life. Once established that stress is here to stay, we began our experimental work.

Starting with the head, we worked our way through the entire body. The issues we addressed in the head included headaches, sinus conditions, and eyestrain. Tension headaches were the major complaint. To relieve headache pain, I recommended slow meditative neck rolls. We proceeded with the exercise and an immediate stilling occurred in the room. These courageous, inquiring first-year med students slowly relaxed and experienced an altered state of consciousness. My heart filled when I looked at these sensitive beings that will be helping to take care of our health concerns in the new millennium.

The next segment of the lecture addressed the use of supplementation. We discussed the use of vitamins, herbs, and homeopathic remedies to relieve stress and to create a more optimal environment. The last and most dramatic part of the lecture had to do with experimental work in which one student acted as the healee and one student acted as the healer. With these healing teams, I instructed the students to sense where energy was needed and to make corrections in the energy fields.

One student had a strong response in her abdomen. She felt a sense of giddiness and lightheadedness. Many students were yawning, which in my opinion can indicate the intense exchange of energy. They tried to be polite and stifle their yawns, but the sleepiness was overwhelming. I explained that this frequently happens when so much energy is circulating.

We discussed the notion of taking care of oneself before attempting to take care of another person. For instance, it is easier and possibly more productive to make sure you are not famished before going in to see a terminally ill cancer patient. Proper nutrition can make you less stressed, more productive, and more present. The idea of "taking a moment" before dashing in to see a patient or dashing to take an exam was discussed. By stopping for a moment, we recalibrate and make ourselves more available for the next situation. Through intelligent self-care the student is able to create a venue that enhances creativity, productivity, intuition, and compassion.

A House Call

One of my students, Alice, was interested in accompanying me on a house call. Helen was expecting us, and at her request we let ourselves in. Helen was seated in a chair looking somewhat forlorn. She had just returned from the hospital after having abdominal surgery, and she was very tired and pale.

Helen has been fully supportive of my work and according to her "tells everyone" about her healer. She was happy to share her experience with a medical student. We stood for a moment and talked to Helen. It felt awkward standing there peering down at her. I suggested that we pull up chairs and have a more comfortable chat. Alice was tense and had the air about her of wanting to do something. The interesting thing about healing is that even though you do something, you almost act as if you were doing nothing. We talked for a few minutes, and the ambiance in the room changed. I sat across from Helen and became aware of an area in the back of her neck that needed attention.

Alice asked what I was doing and I explained to her that I felt as if I could see the back of Helen's neck as I faced her. After I placed my hands on the back of her neck, I invited Alice to touch Helen's neck so that she could feel the imbalance. Her doubting fingers needed to explore before she could feel the imbalance, and then she acknowledged a slight bulge on the left side of Helen's neck.

Alice appeared to be mesmerized by the experience, and at the same time the questions continued. How do you see? What do you look for? How is the energy transferred to Helen? I only had some of the answers and I explained that some scientists are of the opinion that healers are surrounded by vibrational fields that have different frequencies. When these frequencies are transmitted to the healer distresses may begin to resolve.

I continued to work on Helen. After about fifteen minutes, it felt appropriate to have Helen lie on her back. We assisted her to her den and made her comfortable as she lay on her back on her sofa. Helen seemed congested in her abdomen, and I asked if I could lightly place my hand on her abdomen. She said that she was a little tender and that the bloating was still a problem for her. Pressing my hand on her abdomen and her lower back seemed to do the trick. She responded almost immediately; her entire body began to relax. Her hands and forearms had been tense because she had been clutching a pillow to her abdomen. Now they were relaxed and her hands were beginning to warm. Her color was also improved, and the slight smile that came across her face was a very peaceful one.

Interestingly enough during this entire time, Alice was also experiencing some changes. She too was appearing to be more relaxed. As she assisted me, it became obvious that she was becoming more focused and less internally active. When she held Helen's feet she and Helen could both feel energy moving through Alice's fingertips. We moved the energy throughout Helen's body, moving from her feet to the top of her head. At the end of the session, Helen was thoroughly relaxed. She had no pain in her abdomen and I was able to press deeply into her abdomen with my fingers.

Alice was impressed with the results of this session, and we discussed Helen's progress over dinner. I tried to answer her questions about techniques, demographics, and my background. It was an enlightening experience for me to share this time with Alice. She seemed sincerely interested in the work, and it appeared as if she were convinced that these techniques were useful adjuncts to medical procedure.

During a subsequent class, the students learned how to bring energy to their hands. The technique consisted of moving the hands in an exceedingly slow fashion. This slow movement allows energy to move to the hands, and the students were able to experience a tingling and heat in their hands. Using the energy from the hands, we worked on each other.

The students were in relaxed, meditative states and were surprised that time passed so quickly. They were intrigued with the experience and looked radiant by the end of the class.

I have included one student's account of this experience as well as his overall impression of the course:

I initially chose this course because the description reminded me of a type of healing that occurs in Mexican culture. There are people called "sovadores" within our neighborhoods that massage and heal strains, aches, and pains. The course description mentioned similar ailments that the instructor could treat but did not describe the methods used. I enrolled in the course with an open heart and mind, and although it was not what I expected, it provided me with a new awareness and appreciation of alternative healing.

The class began with an introduction to healing energy and its ability to cause cellular transformations. Although interesting, my scientific ears made me skeptical and unsure of the value of our instruction. Despite the worried looks on the students' faces, Dr. Kaye confidently continued with her lecture. Nearing the end of our first session, she wanted to give a class demonstration, so she asked if there was anything bothering us. Fortunately, the previous day I had overexerted myself working out and my arms were unwillingly bent with soreness. Dr. Kaye explained that with little effort she would infuse energy into me, causing a cellular transformation and a relief of my pain. To my surprise, after working ten seconds on one arm, the pain went away. With slightly less skepticism and much more attention placed on any sensations, I asked her to treat my other arm. Again, unexplainably, the pain went away. From this first meeting, and throughout the eight weeks, Dr. Kaye continuously asked (about) our feeling, thoughts, and sensations. This experience and the observations that followed helped diminish my skepticism.

The following meeting, we learned how to feel energy within ourselves and channel this energy to our hands. This also was a unique experience. We lowered the lights and concentrated on moving our arms in a particular pattern while feeling the energy between our hands. During this session, I again kept an open mind and tried to comply with Gloria's instruction. I must admit that I did feel something. My hands felt like they were two magnets repelling each other and I could feel a "center" within my palms. We did this exercise for quite some time, and despite any true sensations, I tried to explain these feeling to myself as arm fatigue.

Although I was still skeptical, something besides curiosity kept me interested in the course.

In the following sessions, Gloria brought in several of her patients. We heard first hand the opinions of people who put their whole confidence into Gloria's healing ability. They shared their stories of the search to find something or someone that could help them deal with the pain of their ailments. In addition to Gloria's healing ability, I now learned that her patient interaction alone must have had some influence in their recovery. I finally discovered that her patient communication skills were what kept me interested in the course. The special interactions that Gloria had with her patients were something that they really needed but could not find with their treating physicians.

The next session, Gloria taught us a technique using energy centers called "Chakras" to help us develop our intuition in using our healing ability. We learned by treating each other and working to move the energy back and forth from head to feet. It was almost like brushing the warm air emitted from the body and moving it away from the center. Here we gained much more confidence, and Gloria and I eventually treated the other medical student with recurring migraine headaches. We all knew that her headaches were very severe, lasted long, and had an almost daily reoccurrence. Yet for the next month, she excitingly reported experiencing only one slight pain for a few minutes. This session was the transition point from skepticism to fascination.

Our final meeting was a site visit at Cedars-Sinai Medical Center. Here we met a plastic surgeon that volunteered his time removing tattoos. Our task was to use our healing touch training to treat the patients before and after the laser treatment. The patients were troubled juveniles trying to turn a new page in their lives by starting a whole new lifestyle. We explained ourselves to the group, and they were willing to participate, so we took them aside in pairs to get treatment. Up to this point things seemed to go as planned, until I began my treatment of one of the teenage boys. The fact that I was a man understandably made the boy uncomfortable. This is where the healing encounter ended. He then requested that one of the girls do the massaging and from then on, the healing touch was transformed in muscle-knot-removing therapy. At the end of the day, something very positive still came out of this visit. We spoke to the plastic surgeon about his opinions on Gloria's work and her involvement in medicine. He said that many of his patients had been frequently asking for something "natural" to help them with the pain of the surgeries. After he would mention Gloria's service they would anxiously want her to be part of the treatment team and would ask how they could get HMOs to pay for it.

Gloria's course accomplished many important goals that made this course one of the most complete learning experiences. She began by convincing us of her healing abilities. Then she showed us that we also could heal. Next she gave examples of people that definitely needed this type of treatment. And finally she showed us why it was important for medical students to learn of the many forms of alternative medicine and their applications within the medical field.

By the time the final semester rolled around, I was confident with my ability to articulate and communicate the subtleties of energetic healing. These students were particularly inquisitive, and over the three-year period that I had been teaching, the interest, intrigue, and acceptance of alternative healing increased. This class was intended for first-year medical students, but in fact a fourth-year student dropped in as did a practicing physician.

The structure remained the same and included lecture, demonstration, experiential opportunities, and patients who had been helped by energetic healing.

During this semester one of the students broke his wrist during a football practice. His break was extensive, and he was in a great deal of pain. I was touched when one of his fellow students interrupted my lecture with a request to help him with his pain.

Another interesting situation occurred when Fox News decided to feature this class on the 11 o'clock news. The students were cooperative and revealing about the impact of the class. One student stated that she thought it would make her a more compassionate physician.

At the end of the class several students summarized their experiences:

> *I have really enjoyed this course. I came into it wanting to broaden my own awareness, wanting to appreciate this mode of healing that so many find effective. I think I am coming away from the course with a more broad, accepting perspective as a healer.*
>
> *Let's see. Coming to class every week was sometimes very tough. Through the week I would become accustomed to the straightforward, logical, black-and-white rhythm of medical*

school. I would become comfortable in the Western system where every question had an answer. Come Thursday, a part of me would struggle and strain against coming to a forum where so little was understood. It was rough to lay my books aside and reach for my own intuition, to stretch my mind around concepts and questions that laughed at logic. It was tough to make myself just flow.

But fortunately, I would muster my will and come. And once here, I never regretted it. I cannot deny that I came away from each class period profoundly relaxed, with a rise in energy. No matter how long the day, or how stressful the week, in this class I found the tensions melting away. I cannot deny that taking the time to connect with myself and my classmates left me feeling healthier. The effect may not have been dramatic every time, but overall, I think that tapping into the need for touch and energy has left me with a great sense of peace.

I have really enjoyed sharing this journey with my classmates. I think we all came in a bit skeptical, more or less. But everyone in the course, in their own way, was able to absorb and appreciate what went on here. I really think highly of the students who, more skeptical than I, were able to set aside their doubts, opening their minds to learn.

So do I have the healing touch? I do believe that when I am focused, and carrying good intention, my touch can raise people's energy. Unfortunately, I don't feel that my touch is extremely powerful—but I think that I can cultivate it by training in massage at some point. People respond in a very real way to human contact, and I want to be able to bring that to people around me. In the course, my favorite was when *we worked on each other. Especially nice was the half hour at the end of class to be worked on by Gloria. Thanks for a great course.*

My experience at UCLA gave me immeasurable hope for the future. At first I was concerned that the lack of documentation in my presentation would invalidate my lectures. In fact, I suspect that my heartfelt presentations were refreshing. Not one student challenged me in any way that made me feel uncomfortable. I was asked some difficult questions, but none were asked with a lack of respect or a negative challenge.

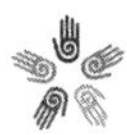

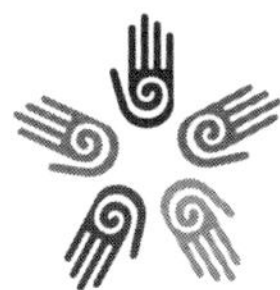

C h a p t e r   1 1

Small Moments

I would like to offer some guidelines that have helped me along the way. Some of these concepts I have gleaned and other notions have been given to me by a number of very wise individuals.

1. Regarding Relationships

In all relationships, whether they are of the same sex, the opposite sex, friends, or foes, the only person or element in the relationship that you can change is yourself. Think for a moment about a difficult relationship you may be having. Can you see how a change in your attitude changes the relationship?

2. Regarding Decisions

A wise friend commented, "Make a decision, and if that doesn't work make another one." Conflict can cause a type of inertia. The self-talk of conflict is very unreliable. When I get into these states, I feel like I am watching a tennis match, only there is no winner or loser. The ball just goes back and forth. Once I make a decision, I usually feel a release from the confusion of indecision. However, I have come to realize that making a decision to do nothing, or to postpone action, is also a decision.

3. Regarding Anger

A wise man gave me wonderful advice when I asked him where anger comes from. He said, "Anger comes from lack of understanding." The more clarity that one has about a situation, the less likely one will experience intense anger. Sometimes having a better understanding about early trauma helps one to understand the present challenge.

4. Regarding Control

Another small moment has to do with a timeline for projects and events. When I was a graduate student, I taught ten yoga classes a week. Since then I have always tried to document the efficacy of esoteric interventions. I was always administering standardized psychological tests to my students. I wanted to demonstrate among other things how yoga practice can affect psychological states. At one time I had four research projects going on simultaneously. Things weren't happening fast enough to suit my rhythm. I was very impatient. My colleagues weren't proceeding with enough interest and speed to suit me. I was aggravated and frustrated. I asked my friend, the wise one, how to handle this situation. This is what he said. "When you are in a line of traffic, you can only move as fast as the traffic moves." At the time I thought that was very unsympathetic. The reality of the situation was actually honored by his remark; you can do your homework and give your best effort, but some things are totally out of your control. As a matter of fact, most things are actually out of your control. It is very difficult to try to control outcomes. Does this mean there is no free will? I don't think so. You may be able to influence a situation, but you cannot control a situation.

5. *Regarding Possessions*

My mentor and dear friend, the late Lila Ostermann, used to tell me that the last shirt has no pockets. In our lifetimes we sometimes accumulate "stuff" that we never really needed in the first place. Stuff can give us a false sense of security and "stuff" can also give us pleasure. It is a hard task to find the balance that relates to material possessions. I am not at all opposed to material possessions and yet, if care is not taken, one can easily become overwhelmed by possessions. How many pairs of shoes can you wear at one time? How many watches can you wear at one time, and how many houses can you live in at the same time?

6. *Regarding Order*

When the physical space is less cluttered, the mind has an opportunity to be less cluttered. Think of the last time you couldn't find your car keys. Do you remember your process? You search your personal space. You search the car. You begin to feel worn down looking for these elusive keys. Your anxiety increases. The mind begins to make alternate plans. Will you be canceling some appointments or calling a friend for assistance? The agitation begins to build. It takes over in the mind and body.

The simplicity associated with order can be a great comfort. The mind can retain a focus, and action taken from the vantage point of order and simplicity has a potency of its own.

7. Regarding Life's Challenges

Another wise man once told me that every moment is perfect. I had difficulty believing this at the time. I was in the throes of experiencing a very difficult time when my friend gave me his words of wisdom. I thought that he was exceedingly insensitive, and I didn't really understand that he was trying to comfort me with his words. When you begin to think of life and its challenges as an institution of very higher learning, the perfection of the moment begins to make some sense. We don't always get to choose the moments, but that doesn't make them less perfect.

8. Regarding Being Present; Not Perfect

Be present; not perfect. So many of us have been programmed to perform in a certain way. We expect a certain performance from ourselves and others. Sitting with someone who is troubled is a true gift. This is not the time to fix things or take action; rather, it is a time for being, not doing.

9. Regarding Attitude

Develop an attitude of gratitude. Resentment, anger, jealousy, and fear reduce an ability to develop an attitude of gratitude. When life's irritations cause us to react with negativity we diminish our ability to be in the present. Unresolved issues frequently play a part in this negativity. An attitude of gratitude truly accepts what is happening in the present. You accept challenge, adversity, joy, and pleasure. It all becomes the same.

10. Regarding Challenge

Powerful people get powerful lessons. Many powerful people put themselves in positions so that they are unwittingly brought to their knees. The difficulty with powerful people is that more often than not, they believe that they can handle the situation put in front of them. Therefore, their lessons can be even more powerful and challenging.

11. Regarding Effective Effort

Be absolutely alert and make no effort. This notion comes directly from the spiritual leader, Krishamurti. Line up your ducks. Do some homework and wait for an outcome. The waiting for me can be the most challenging aspect of this instruction. It is a definite task to do the work and line up the ducks. It is an indefinite task to wait and watch the fruits of your labor unfold. This waiting period can be frustrating and awkward, but have patience.

12. Regarding the Status of the Ego

You have to have an ego before you can give it up. In my opinion, an inflated ego is as challenging as a deflated one. The individual who spouts ideas of grandiosity lacks an ego integration. A similar but converse situation is the individual who continually thinks that belittling oneself is an act of humility. The grandiose individual has ideas of an unrealistic magnitude. The identified humble servant is in all probability the individual who has a "poor me" attitude.

13. Regarding the Non-Existence of the Perfect Wave

Much of life can be wasted waiting for the perfect wave. When we wait for the perfect moment or the perfect opportunity or the perfect condition we are frequently immobilized and take no action. This stagnant state in which there is no action or movement can create an uncomfortable paralysis. With the knowledge that there is no perfect wave one can step forward and initiate informed action.

14. Regarding Non-Violence

When one thinks of non-violence it is obvious that physical violence, abuse, destruction, and killing are violent acts. What is not as obvious is violent thought directed at oneself. The self-talk can take over and be very destructive.

Self-talk such as "I am not good enough," "Nobody likes me," "I'm unattractive," or "I'm stupid," are all examples of destructive violent thought. The fact that it is self-directed, in my opinion, is more destructive than it would be if it were directed by someone else. If you, in fact, direct these violent thoughts towards yourself, your only real recourse is to stop the thought process. This is a much more difficult task. When you are able to stop these thoughts, you become much more gentle with yourself. The self-acceptance that you begin to experience is a delight in itself.

15. Regarding Truthfulness

There are so many considerate ways to be truthful. Rather than to be offensive and abusively truthful, I have found the phrase "that doesn't work for me" to cover much ground. If someone tries to engage you in conversation and the topic is a sensitive one, it is inoffensive and truthful to say, "That topic is not open for discussion."

Another aspect of truthfulness is being truthful with oneself. It is sometimes hard to see the truth. Am I being true to myself? Am I walking my talk? Am I speaking the truth? How clear is my assessment of this situation?

16. Regarding Presence

The importance of being present cannot be overrated. A distraction, a hidden agenda, and a reluctance to face reality are all means to take us away from being present. In a relationship being present can enable participants to more clearly hear each other. Being in the moment helps one to be present. In life being in the moment and having an awareness of that state eases emotional reactions.

§

I hope that these small moments may be valuable for you; I certainly have been guided by these concepts.

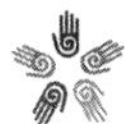

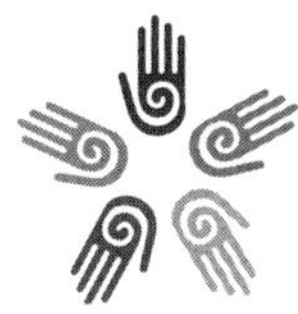

Chapter 12

Summary

Healing is a very complex, yet simple business. My former guru wrote me a letter in the mid-seventies. He said that you can learn many therapeutic techniques, but the greatest teacher is love. I have not specifically addressed love as such, but I have talked about ego and staying out of the healing process by being as clear a channel as possible. The term unconditional love is frequently mentioned in New Age literature. My difficulty with this concept is that we are mere mortals, and in my opinion, incapable of unconditional loving. We may think that we are giving freely, but when we have expectations or intentions we are not as free as we think we are.

I certainly try to do the best that I can and stay out of my own way, but certain conditions and life experiences touch me more deeply than others. I am particularly attached to outcome when children need treatment. I am also deeply touched when someone has a very strong belief that I can help them. I need to watch my ego and not be charmed by someone else's belief system.

The most loving, selfless and powerful person I have ever met was a true Guru named Kripalvananda. He spoke no English and when he came to this country he continued his vow of silence. He communicated his thoughts by writing them on a chalkboard. He maintained his vocal chords by chanting. He was the most evolved human being I have ever met. When his time came to pass, his body did not go into rigor mortis for several days. Even though he had passed, the energy continued to move through him.

By observation he taught me about vulnerability and ego. In his later years, his long fasts caused him to appear vulnerable. I watched him maneuver a wooden staircase. He slowly groped his way down the single flight of steps. His disciples were behind him not in front of him. I was appalled as I viewed this from a distance. The disciples were being respectful but were not protecting him. My lesson was to see that the more vulnerable an individual is, the less vulnerable that individual is. To be truly open, one experiences life with less fear and fewer expectations. It was a very valuable lesson to observe and a very difficult one to live.

This notion of vulnerability and openness is important in the healing interaction. Without expectations, the energy may move more efficiently through you and you become a clearer channel for your client. Being present and passively alert creates a potent space for healing. In this stillness, the vibrations can almost become palpable. The intermingling of energy fields become a loving embrace that potentiates healing of the body, mind and spirit.

§

I've now shared with you the very basic techniques of healing. I would like to leave you with five very important notions.

1. The energy has a far higher intelligence than you do.
   Many times I place my hands on what seems like an area unrelated to the complaint. Because of the amazing intelligence of the energy, the healing follows. The energy just seems to know where to go and what to do. Trusting the energy is part of the process.

2. Beware of the ego. This is not a power trip.
   It is important to have ego so that you can let it go. However, if you are seduced into thinking that your ego is important, you face the possibility of entertaining a power trip. This is a no-win situation for you, nor anyone you are attempting to help.

3. You are being used as a conduit for healing energy. You are not the healing energy.
   Be a clear channel for the energy; let it move naturally. Do not over-think the process.

4. Be lighthearted as you experience this profound phenomenon.
   Healing is a beautiful phenomenon. Caress it with gratitude and in a loving, lighthearted way.

5. Serve, surrender, and love.
   This concept is a blueprint for life. When you serve – you help another, when you surrender—you are in the moment and accepting, and when you love—your heart opens to give and receive. Is there a more beautiful gift?

"My name is Lucy Prieto; Dr. Kaye has treated my little dog, my son, my daughter, my son-in-law, my daughter-in-law, my grand-sons, and myself. She is our go-to healer when we need any kind of help.

"People just can't go wrong when they go see Dr. Kaye. She was born with the gift; no matter what is troubling you, you will walk away feeling better."

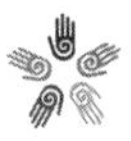

www.DrGloriaKaye.com